19-99.

Early Psychosocial Interventions in Dementia

of related interest

Depression in Later Life
Jill Manthorpe and Steve Iliffe
ISBN 978 1 84310 234 2

Involving Families in Care Homes
A Relationship-Centred Approach to Dementia Care
Bob Woods, John Keady and Diane Seddon
ISBN 978 1 84310 229 8
Bradford Dementia Group Good Practice Guides

The Pool Activity Level (PAL) Instrument for Occupational Profiling
A Practical Resource for Carers of People with Cognitive Impairment
3rd edition
Jackie Pool
ISBN 978 1 84310 594 7
Bradford Dementia Group Good Practice Guides

Design for Nature in Dementia Care
Garuth Chalfont
ISBN 978 1 84310 571 8
Bradford Dementia Group Good Practice Guides

How to Make Your Care Home Fun
Simple Activities for People of All Abilities
Kenneth Agar
ISBN 978 1 84310 952 5

Remembering Yesterday, Caring Today
Reminiscence in Dementia Care: A Guide to Good Practice
Pam Schweitzer and Errollyn Bruce
Foreword by Faith Gibson
ISBN 978 1 84310 649 4
Bradford Dementia Group Good Practice Guides

Early Psychosocial Interventions in Dementia

Evidence-Based Practice

Edited by Esme Moniz-Cook
and Jill Manthorpe

Jessica Kingsley Publishers
London and Philadelphia

First published in 2009
by Jessica Kingsley Publishers
116 Pentonville Road
London N1 9JB, UK
and
400 Market Street, Suite 400
Philadelphia, PA 19106, USA

www.jkp.com

Library of Congress Cataloging in Publication Data
Psychosocial interventions in early dementia : evidence-based practice / edited by Esme Moniz-Cook and Jill Manthorpe.
      p. ; cm.
      Includes bibliographical references.
      ISBN 978-1-84310-683-8 (pb : alk. paper)
      1. Dementia--Patients--Care--Europe. 2. Evidence-based medicine--Europe. I. Moniz-Cook, Esme. II. Manthorpe, Jill, 1955-
      [DNLM: 1. Dementia--psychology--Europe. 2. Evidence-Based Medicine--Europe. 3. Psychotherapy--methods--Europe. WM 220 P9745 2009]
      RC521.P79 2009
      616.89--dc22
                        2008024649

British Library Cataloguing in Publication Data
A CIP catalogue record for this book is available from the British Library

ISBN 978 1 84310 683 8

Printed and bound in Great Britain by
Athenaeum Press, Gateshead, Tyne and Wear

Contents

List of Illustrations   7

Acknowledgements   9

1   **Introduction: Personalising Psychosocial Interventions to Individual Needs and Context**   11
Esme Moniz-Cook and Jill Manthorpe

PART I   SUPPORT AT THE TIME OF DIAGNOSIS   37

2   **What Do We Tell People with Dementia about Their Diagnosis and How Do We Tell Them?**   39
Hilary J. Husband

3   **Timely Psychosocial Interventions in a Memory Clinic**   50
Esme Moniz-Cook, Gillian Gibson, Jas Harrison and Hannah Wilkinson

PART II   COGNITIVE AND MEMORY SUPPORT   71

4   **Working with Memory Problems: Cognitive Rehabilitation in Early Dementia**   73
Linda Clare

5   **Cognitive Stimulation for People with Mild Cognitive Impairment and Early Dementia**   81
Inge Cantegreil-Kallen, Jocelyne de Rotrou and Anne-Sophie Rigaud

6   **GRADIOR: A Personalised Computer-based Cognitive Training Programme for Early Intervention in Dementia**   93
Manuel Franco, Kate Jones, Bob Woods and Pablo Gomez

7   **Memory Groups for People with Early Dementia**   106
Molly Burnham

8   Health Technologies for People with   115
     Early Dementia: The ENABLE Project
     Suzanne Cahill, Emer Begley and Inger Hagen

**PART III   PSYCHOLOGICAL, EMOTIONAL   133
AND SOCIAL SUPPORT**

9   Group Psychotherapy for People with   135
     Early Dementia
     Richard Cheston

10   Art Therapy: Getting in Touch with Inner Self   146
     and Outside World
     Steffi Urbas

11   A Host of Golden Memories: Individual   156
     and Couples Group Reminiscence
     Irene Carr, Karen Jarvis and Esme Moniz-Cook

12   Developing Group Support for Men with Mild   174
     Cognitive Difficulties and Early Dementia
     Jill Manthorpe and Esme Moniz-Cook

13   Group Psycho-Educational Intervention   186
     for Family Carers
     Rabih Chattat, Marie V. Gianelli
     and Giancarlo Savorani

**PART IV   DEVELOPING EVIDENCE-BASED   199
PSYCHOSOCIAL SUPPORT SERVICES**

14   The Meeting Centres Support Programme   201
     Rose-Marie Dröes, Franka Meiland, Jacomine de Lange,
     Myrra Vernooij-Dassen and Willem van Tilburg

15   Personalised Disease Management for   211
     People with Dementia: The Primary
     Carer Support Programme
     Myrra Vernooij-Dassen, Maud Graff
     and Marcel Olde Rikkert

16   Carer Interventions in the Voluntary Sector   222
     Georgina Charlesworth, Joanne Halford,
     Fiona Poland and Susan Vaughan

     List of Contributors   230
     Index   234

LIST OF ILLUSTRATIONS

Tables

1.1	National circumstances: epidemiology and mental health facilities	12
1.2	Guidelines for choosing psychosocial intervention	30
5.1	Contents of a Cognitive Stimulation session	84
8.1	Description of assistive devices being tested in Ireland	119
8.2	Socio-demographic and cognitive characteristics of people with dementia	121
8.3	Use of products reported by person with dementia six months after devices were installed	121
8.4	Carers' perceptions of use of products by their care recipient six months after installation	122
8.5	Carers' own use of assistive devices six months after installation	123
8.6	People with dementia – usefulness of assistive devices six months after installation	124
8.7	Carers' perceptions of usefulness of assistive devices for person with dementia six months after installation	124
11.1	Results of Autobiographical Memory Interview (AMI) scores	168
13.1	Change over time on relevant outcome measures	193
16.1	Pre- and post-group mean scores (standard deviation) for 24 participant carers	225

Figures

3.1	Using a simplified 'cognitive map' to discuss the memory assessment	59
3.2	Example of written information provided for Fleur and her family	60
6.1	Effect of GRADIOR on Paula	103
8.1	Pictorial examples of the assistive technologies evaluated in Ireland	120
10.1	'Without Words'	149
10.2	Angela's 'mandalas'	150
10.3	The priest's holidays	152
11.1	Harold's collage	164
14.1	The programme and its goals	206

Boxes

1.1	Illustrations of individually desired outcomes	25
3.1	Family workshop: 'Understanding and Coping with Memory as You Get Older'	56
6.1	Overcoming practical obstacles to the application of neuropsychological rehabilitation programmes in dementia	96
6.2	Example of how the GRADIOR system works	99
6.3	Adam and his wife: rehabilitation with GRADIOR	101
6.4	Paula – intervention with GRADIOR	102
7.1	Topics covered on memory group therapy course	109
7.2	An example of a course handout	110
12.1	Background of three men in one group	178
12.2	What would you like from these group sessions?	183
12.3	The importance of wives	183
15.1	Questions for carers and potential strategies	215

Acknowledgements

Our sincere thanks to Linda Clare for initial help with manuscript preparation, staff at the Hull Memory Clinic, UK, for ongoing support over the past decade, Margaret Bowes and especially Clare Wilder for assistance in updating chapters. We also sincerely thank Alison Greenley and Andrew Walker for their dedicated patience and assistance in bringing this work to completion. Some of the material in this book was co-funded by the Commission of European Communities with The University of Hull, UK, Hull and Holderness Community Health NHS Trust (now Humber Mental Health Teaching NHS Trust) UK, and the Eastern Health Board, Dublin, Ireland, between 1 December 1997 and 1 December 1999 – *FILE NO: SOC 97 201452 05F03 'Early Detection and Psychosocial Rehabilitation to Maintain Quality of Life – A Training Package in Dementia'* and we thank them for this early support.

We thank members of *INTERDEM* for their continuing inspiration and collegiality, especially the authors of the chapters in this book. This book is dedicated to the people with dementia and their supporters across Europe who have permitted us to tell part of their stories and shared their experiences. In all cases described we have used pseudonyms. The cover of this book has been reproduced from the case material in Chapter 11 (figure 11.1), first developed as training materials for the use of collage in early stage dementia by Karen Jarvis (Community Mental health Nurse) as part of the Queens Nursing Institute and the Alzheimer's Society Fund for Innovation: Excellence in Dementia Care Nursing Award.

Chapter 1

Introduction: Personalising Psychosocial Interventions to Individual Needs and Context

**Esme Moniz-Cook
and Jill Manthorpe**

Overview

This book describes the emerging evidence base for psychosocial interventions in dementia care. It uses examples from practitioners and researchers working in a range of settings across Europe. This first chapter makes the case for developing pan-European psychosocial interventions to support older people with suspected or early dementia and their families. It then outlines how the interventions described in subsequent chapters can be personalised to individual concerns and contexts. Four areas of early intervention are considered:

- at the time of diagnosis

- cognition and memory-oriented support

- psychological and social support

- service developments within which these interventions can be based.

The chapter concludes with a stepped care framework for psychosocial intervention in early dementia.

Table 1.1 National circumstances: epidemiology and mental health facilities (*source: www.who.int/mental_health)

EU country	Incidence of dementia	Prevalence of dementia	*Percentage of health budget to gross domestic product (GDP)	*Percentage of health budget on mental health expenditure	*Number of specialist medical professionals per 100,000 population (where known)
The Netherlands	Age 55+ 9.8/1000 (Ruitenberg et al. 2001) Males 10.5: Females 17.3 (Launer et al. 1999)	Total: Age 55+ 6.3% (Ott et al. 1995)	8.8	7	Psychiatrists 9 Psychologists 28 Neurologists 3.7
Belgium	Age 60+ 0.53 (Buntinx et al. 2002)	Age 65+ 6–9% (Vlief et al. 2002)	8	6	Psychiatrists 18 Psychologists Neurologists 1
UK	Males 10.7 Females 18.5 (Launer et al. 1999)	Ages 65–70 1 in 50 Ages 70–80 1 in 20 Ages 80+ 1 in 5 (Alzheimer's Society website)	5.8	10	Psychiatrists 11 Psychologists 9 Neurologists 1
Spain	No information available	Total: Age 65+ 5 (Lobo et al. 1995)–16% (Vilalta-Franch et al. 2000)	8	No information available	Psychiatrists 3.6 Psychologists 1.9 Neurologists 2.5
Italy	150.000 new cases per year (Di Carlo et al. 2002)	Males 5.3% Ages 65–84 Females 7.2% Ages 65–84 (Ilsa 1997)	9.3	No information available	Psychiatrists 9 Psychologists 3 Neurologists
Portugal	No information available	No information available	8.2	No information available	Psychiatrists 5 Psychologists 2.8 Neurologists 2.3
France	Males 11.5 Females 15.2 (Launer et al. 1999) 165.000 new cases per year (Ramaroson et al. 2003)	Age 65+ 5% (Ramaroson et al. 2003) 800.000 prevalent cases ≥ 75: 18 % (Ramaroson et al. 2003)	9.8	5	Psychiatrists 20 Psychologists Neurologists
Ireland	4000 new cases per year (Keogh and Roche 1996)	Age 65+: 5.5% (Keogh and Roche 1996)	6.2	7.7	Psychiatrists 5 Psychologists 9.7 Neurologists 0.4

Taken from Vernooij-Dassen et al. (2005).

Rationale for this book

Dementia is a major problem of later life for many, although not all, older people. As the population ages, demand for support services is likely to increase dramatically. The complexity of the needs of people with dementia and their carers presents challenges across Europe (see Table 1.1), exposing the lack of co-ordinated approaches to policy and the limited attention by professionals and services to meeting people's needs for support and care in most states (Warner *et al.* 2002).

There is little for practitioners in the way of internationally accepted evidence-based psychosocial interventions for people with early dementia, since, not only is evidence-based practice in psychosocial intervention difficult to achieve (Woods 2003), but where it exists studies have understandably concentrated on the difficulties of care when the person's symptoms may be severe and disabling (Parahoo, Campbell and Scoltock 2002). Thus, most dementia care intervention literature relates to family carer 'burden', nursing home care or drug therapy. As we shall see in the chapters of this book, this does not mean that there is no evidence for psychosocial intervention in early dementia since, in an overview on the subject, Woods (2003) concludes that: 'as with many other fields of research, probably the biggest question is how to implement widely what has already been identified as good, evidence-based practice' (p.6).

There are at least four reasons for the lack of widespread knowledge of the emerging evidence base for early psychosocial intervention in dementia care, particularly on what can be offered to people with dementia themselves. We shall consider each of these and outline how this book may help to address these gaps in current knowledge and associated practice.

First, is the belief that local or national contexts are unique and that knowledge and practice is not translatable, with a tendency for practitioners to confine themselves to their own local or national contexts. This book challenges this perspective and seeks to reduce the current reliance on a few passionate champions, valuable as they are, to spur change in dementia care. There are, indeed, growing opportunities for practitioners across Europe to learn from services that are embedded within national health and social care systems that have been working beyond experimental or project status for some time. We suggest that there is much to learn from each other across nations and that practitioners in English-speaking countries such as the UK may often miss opportunities to explore intervention and support in dementia care that have developed throughout mainland Europe. Taking a pan-European perspective reveals the richness of psychosocial support in practice and potentially offers much to learn of what works and what does not. Despite the nation-specific cultures, different models of health and social care services, diverse languages, varying professional roles and funding routes (Vernooij-Dassen *et al.* 2005), European states are a fertile arena in which to explore how people with dementia at an early stage can be supported to enhance their quality of life and well-being.

Second, is a weakness in research and practice in dementia care since this has, understandably, concentrated on the position of family carers. Whilst the needs of families are highly relevant to Europe, especially in states where family and female kin shoulder most caregiving responsibilities (Cameron and Moss 2007), this perspective has until recently tended to obscure the potential for psychosocial support for people themselves, including what they may need to understand and manage the day-to-day consequences of living with a dementia. Apart from the concluding chapters of this book in Part IV, where services are described as a context within which older people with early dementia may be supported, the focus of most chapters is weighted towards the support of people with dementia. However, given the family caregiving literature which suggests that the most effective psychosocial interventions are those that include both the person with dementia and their family carer (Brodaty, Green and Koschera 2003), we have made the assumption that most psychosocial interventions, whether directed at the person or the family 'carer',[1] inevitably have to take into account all aspects of supportive systems including the person and primary 'carer', the wider family and supporting friends.

Third, is the definitional issue of early dementia, because this is where biomedical or clinical processes associated with early detection, recognition and diagnosis often compete with practice and research in psychosocial intervention and/or rehabilitation. Unlike the former, the latter has its roots in attention to individual differences, theories of personality and human motivation, identity theory, life span psychology, social psychology and relationships, all of which guide the growth and targeting of psychosocial interventions. They are also influenced by social construction approaches that affect the wider context of services for people with dementia.

Most of the interventions and services described in this book are for older people and their families, since it is this age group that most generally experiences emerging or newly recognised dementia – referred to for ease as *early dementia*. Early or newly diagnosed dementia is an area where services are increasingly needed to meet the rising interests and other policy developments. Having a diagnosis of dementia is only the start of the process of recognition and the potential for a 'care gap' (Iliffe and Manthorpe 2004) may emerge, when people are left with a diagnosis but little support during the early stages of their dementia. A partial exception to this is, of course, where licensing of the anti-dementia drugs in early dementia has driven whole systems of support for those who are eligible for drug therapy. For example, in the UK and Ireland, a recent textbook for community mental health nurses (Keady, Clarke and Page 2007) opens its section on professional practice with issues surrounding Alzheimer's medication (Beavis 2007) and nurse prescribing (Page 2007). The hope and optimism brought to dementia care for people, families and practitioners through drug therapy developments remain an important opportunity when these early intervention medication services also adopt a public health promotion component (Beavis 2007, pp.111–112). However, these often have developed: 'on an ad-hoc basis, rather than by following a defined evidence based protocol' (p.112).

Some commentators suggest that in terms of resource allocation the prevailing disease model of dementia and associated pharmacological approaches compete unfairly with other forms of support that may be important to people with dementia (Heller and Heller 2003). This may be one reason for poorly conceived and ad hoc development of proactive health promotion and psychosocial interventions. Chapter 3 of this book outlines a primary care based psychosocial intervention (incorporating a health promotion component) in a memory clinic. This was evaluated in an exploratory randomised controlled trial, prior to the widespread introduction of the anti-dementia (acetylchoninestrase inhibitor, AChEI) drugs in the UK.

Many governments stress the importance of early detection in their dementia strategies to help prepare individuals and their carers (Moise et al. 2004) and in the UK this is a focus of the National Dementia Strategy (to be published late 2008). Timely recognition of dementia might have different expressions across Europe owing to national variations in priorities, resources, service patterns and professional cultures. However, practitioners face similar problems in supporting increasing numbers of people with newly diagnosed dementia and making a reality of the advantages of early recognition.

A fourth reason for lack of knowledge of what can be done to support older people with early dementia themselves relates to what has come to be known as the 'double stigma' of age and dementia (Benbow and Reynolds 2000). For example, many of the interventions outlined in the chapters of this book were documented in DIADEM, a pan-European study of dementia in eight European states, where it was noted that irrespective of dementia resources, the stigma associated with dementia was an overriding factor in many countries and seemed to explain the lack of supportive interventions or underuse of these where they existed (Vernooij-Dassen et al. 2005). This finding sets the interventions described in this book within an explanatory context. We suggest that developing practice or services is not a simple matter of arguing that the evidence for their benefits is robust, or that such interventions have the potential to work alongside pharmacological treatments, or that there is scope for these when pharmacological treatment is not possible. In addition, practitioners and service developers need to address the stigma of dementia in their approaches to supporting older people with suspected dementia and their families. In our view, stigma is a powerful explanation for why, despite the small but sound emerging evidence for psychosocial support, services for people with early dementia remain underdeveloped or underused. Furthermore, the construct of stigma affects not only people with dementia but also those associated with this disability, including families, other supporters and health and social care professionals.

Understanding stigma in dementia

Stigma is a social construct which can underpin biomedical constructs of age and dementia in health and social care provision. Older people with dementia have to overcome the double stigma of age and dementia, both of which inevitably affect the quality of their lives, the services that support them and the national policies that underpin these services.

Three types of stigma, reflecting a process of disqualification whereby a 'normal' person is reduced to a person with whom something is wrong, were conceptualised by Goffman (1963) and each of these can be understood in the context of dementia. The first relates to differences of the physical human body and appearances, such as physical impairments or disabilities. For example, older people with suspected dementia and their families often associated dementia with inevitable difficulties with mobility and loss of control of vital body functions (Moniz-Cook *et al.* 2006). The second relates to the view that an individual has personal 'blemishes' which negatively affect social status. In dementia care, ageism (the view that older people are rigid, inflexible, unable to change), combined with biomedical disease models of dementia as a progressive disease, appears to have fostered the belief among some professionals, such as family doctors across Europe, that nothing can be done in early dementia (Vernooij-Dassen *et al.* 2005); thus perhaps unfairly disqualifying people with dementia from rehabilitation services and resources. This second type of stigma is also seen in the view that having dementia inevitably results in 'madness' – that is, a 'spoiled' social identity. For example, people with suspected dementia and their families at a memory clinic have reported fears of loss of 'mind' and worries about the effects on personal relationships (Moniz-Cook *et al.* 2006). The third type – 'tribal stigma' – refers to the grouping of individuals and negative perceptions of the group. In the present service context groupings occur based on age and cognition. The consequence is a marginalisation of older people with dementia within health and social care systems and also other facilities such as those related to housing, leisure and cultural activities. Tribal stigma in dementia is also seen in the view that people with dementia do not have 'capacity' to make any decisions due to cognitive loss and that decisions must therefore be made for them. Thus, the views of other people, such as family members, are seen as sufficient, and where family carers become distressed, few options for the continued support of the person with dementia in the home exist. One consequence of this is inappropriate and undesired admission to care homes, rather than tailored community-based services of the sort that are increasingly available for and demanded by younger people with disabilities across Europe (Cameron and Moss 2007).

Addressing stigma in early dementia

To summarise the process by which the types of stigma seems to occur in dementia, we suggest that the unifying concept is that of a 'spoiled identity', although this has yet to be fully informed by the views and experiences of people with dementia. A study of the experience of people in the early stages of dementia note that whilst most perceived their quality of life as 'good' and were satisfied with it, many had experienced stigma, which they believed had affected their lives (Katsuno 2005). Furthermore, stigma leading to high internalised shame and low levels of personal control can be particularly marked in dementia in comparison with other neurological impairments (Burgener and Berger 2008). Stigma rests on the belief that there is little to offer people with dementia, since it is a deteriorating disease, leading to a reluctance in making an early diagnosis and pessimism about prognosis, which in turn forges another link in the chain of rehabilitative nihilism – that nothing can be done – in early dementia. Stigma may therefore influence delays in recognition and diagnosis through the processes of concealment, minimisation or the ignoring of early signs and symptoms. Even where a diagnosis of dementia is strongly suspected, stigma and a desire to protect individuals are often cited by professionals as a reason for not disclosing a dementia diagnosis (Bamford *et al.* 2004), particularly since the area is often emotionally highly charged with family fears (Moniz-Cook *et al.* 2006) and potentially influenced by preceding 'protective caregiving' whereby spouses may believe that they are protecting the self-image of their partner with a developing dementia (Gillies 1995). Thus, in the early stages, 'wait and see' or 'wait until it progresses' are commonly held views among older people with suspected dementia, families and many professionals such as family doctors. Furthermore, whether or not an anti-dementia drug is available or relevant, the option for psychosocial intervention may be undermined. Even when pharmacological or drug treatments are used, the 'search for a cure' may obscure family and professional efforts towards psychosocial interventions to minimise the extra or preventable disabilities that are often associated with dementia.

The interventions and services outlined in the chapters of this book address some of the consequences of stigma in early dementia. For example, in line with the growing involvement of people with dementia in public events and services (Clare, Rowlands and Quinn 2008), improved health promotion interventions at an early stage (Chapter 3) provide avenues for counteracting the first type of stigma. Practitioners can also use the time of diagnosis (Chapters 2 and 3) as an opportunity to strengthen personal and social identities for people with early dementia. Some of the interventions outlined in Part III (Chapters 10–12) have further scope in early dementia for strengthening personal and social identities though maintaining valuable family and social relationships. Social stigma associated with dementia that prevents service development has been addressed in the Netherlands (Chapter 15) where there are now well-designed studies of case management of dementia in primary care (Jansen et al. 2005). Developing ongoing timely psychosocial intervention and support for people with dementia from the start (Chapter 3) is a first step towards counteracting 'tribal' stigma. In addition, there are now studies showing that people with dementia living at home and in care homes are capable of learning new information (Chapter 4; Bird 2000; Camp, Bird and Cherry 2000; Clare and Woods 2001) and that they may have 'cognitive reserve' suggesting that the brain may actively attempt to compensate for the challenge represented by damage due to dementia (Stern 2007). These studies continue to challenge the notion, which we suggest has its origins in 'tribal' stigma, that rehabilitation and recovery are not possible in dementia. There is growing evidence (Mittelman, Epstein and Pierzchala 2003; Mittelman et al. 2006; Moniz-Cook et al. 2008a; Chapter 13) and new studies (Joling et al. 2008) showing that families can be trained and supported to maintain their own well-being and minimise distress through timely psychosocial intervention and ongoing support. This offers other practical ways by which 'tribal' stigma and its negative consequences may be reduced for people with dementia.

The similarity of the process and consequences of stigma that we have outlined was striking across all European states that participated in the DIADEM study (Vernooij-Dassen et al. 2005). As noted previously, in most cases this did not seem closely associated with investment in services or availability of professional support. However, the precise nature and processes of stigma across nations remain complex, since stigma attached to dementia is manifested by differences both within and amongst European countries (Iliffe et al. 2005) and by some common themes. For example, the prevailing hesitation surrounding early recognition by family doctors is stronger in some countries such as Spain and Portugal where physicians seem to be particularly wary about providing a diagnosis of dementia (Iliffe *et al.* 2005), whilst in the Netherlands and the UK guidelines exist to help professionals overcome the known obstacles to timely recognition and diagnosis (see NICE/SCIE 2006; SIGN 2006; Wind *et al.* 2003). In some countries, such as Portugal, avoidance of the 'dementia' label is related to resources, since it may limit access to nursing home care (Iliffe *et al.* 2005), whilst in others such as Belgium there is a national and sometimes polarised debate on the rights to refuse treatment or to have it withdrawn, with one view that 'suffering' from dementia reflects an undignified existence and another (predominantly from the Alzheimer societies) that preserving the dignity of people with dementia is an important endeavour. This polarisation may be underpinned by stigmatised public attitudes, since a literature review of the perspective of patients with dementia suggests that they are often active agents in minimising their suffering and coping with the challenges that they face (de Boer *et al.* 2007). In countries where guidelines for professionals have been developed such as the Netherlands (Wind *et al.* 2003), Scotland (SIGN 2006) and England (NICE/SCIE 2006) there is the potential for extracting the necessary detail on the observed variation and its causes which may also offer suggestions about the pattern of services. Developing guidelines for professionals where these do not exist or updating them to address the obstacles to timely diagnosis, for example, as in the Netherlands, are change strategies that can improve professional practice. They can also foster greater debate surrounding the tensions that exist across practice where some desire to minimise harm through avoiding early diagnosis whilst others believe that this conflicts with autonomy and human rights.

The consequence of the double stigma of age and dementia combined with family fears is that practitioners, researchers and students alike quickly realise that working with people with dementia on a day-to-day basis entails personal emotional investment as well as organisational and political skills. This means that they too need support and that this should be part of any service or locality. Attention to increasing public awareness needs to be matched by better support for those working in this area, whether they are part of large organisations or work on their own directly for people with dementia and their families (Breda *et al.* 2006).

The variety and range of innovation, psychosocial practice and service development across Europe are increasingly combined with campaigns to raise public awareness of dementia. In some countries such as the Netherlands, the UK and France, where there are strong Alzheimer societies and disabled people's movements, the power of stigma appears to be decreasing in the general population. Shame associated with having a family member with dementia may also be gradually declining in these countries, with the growing self-confidence of carers' groups, campaigning organisations and people with dementia themselves (Friedell and Bryden-Boden 2002) informing the debate on what is needed. However, practitioners working in mainstream services for people with early dementia will also need to provide leadership if the aspirations for a rapid expansion of early psychosocial interventions are to be realised. Practice developments will need to occur in both specialist teams as well as more generic settings, such as community centres, adult education and primary health and social care.

Well-developed early interventions will be their own ambassadors for addressing stigma and reducing professionals' apprehension about leaving people with a diagnosis, but without support. This book provides examples of such services and it is notable that they do not report any lack of interest or demand for what they offer and reflect much of what people with dementia outline as important in early dementia (Bryden-Boden 2002).

Psychosocial intervention in early dementia

Readers are likely to be familiar with many techniques and services that come under the psychosocial umbrella and may have encountered advocates for many of them. We will briefly describe the interventions that can be broadly classified as psychosocial to set the context for this book. These are wide ranging but all aim to minimise the risks of future disability. They include:

- signposting

- intensive communication methods

- standard psychological therapies

- therapies to promote well-being.

Signposting

Signposting involves alerting a person and the family to an informative website on dementia, or to internet-based support with others across the world, or to the Alzheimer's Society for local information, or to handing out educational information sheets.

Intensive communication methods

These methods include telling people their diagnosis and about the provision of therapeutic support, fostering positive attitudes towards rehabilitation in a person with dementia and their support networks.

Standard psychological therapies

These include cognitive therapy, behaviour therapy, anxiety management and relaxation, psychotherapeutic group work and individual life review, which have shown benefit in reducing distress in people with dementia and their carers (see the overview by Moniz-Cook 2008), where anxiety, depression and conflict are present.

Therapies to promote well-being

Most of the interventions described in this book are concerned not with the treatment of existing distress, but with the prevention of distress and the associated extra disabilities that can ensue. This can be achieved by fostering positive attitudes towards rehabilitation in the person with dementia, the family and other support networks. Some of these psychosocial interventions have been subject to the 'gold standard' of randomised controlled trials or such trials are currently underway. The best known of these that may be applied in early dementia services are: those that promote cognition (i.e. Cognitive Stimulation Therapy, CST; Cognitive Training, CT; and Cognitive Rehabilitation, CR); those that support psychological and social relationships (such as activity-based reminiscence); those that support family carers; and those that support both the person with dementia and the carer. Each of these will be examined next.

Group CST (or what was known as reality orientation) developed its early evidence base in France with subsequent evidence from the UK studies by Spector and her colleagues (www.cstdementia.com/index.php, accessed 2 August 2008) reporting a positive impact on cognition (comparable to published studies of pharmacological studies of the acetylcholinesterase inhibitors) and quality of life (see Moniz-Cook 2006). Studies of individual in-home CST are yet to emerge, although in Italy, Onder and colleagues (2005) used a standardised session-based manual to deliver CST (described as reality orientation) for 30 minutes three times per week over 25 weeks. With recent international interest in the concept of Mild Cognitive Impairment (MCI) and aspirations to offer support to protect against progression to dementia (Tuokko and Hultsch 2006), application of group-based CST to people with MCI has been described by the team at Broca Hospital, France (Chapter 5). The notion of cognition as a muscle that requires exercise (i.e. CT) has become a popular method of trying to reduce the risk of dementia, attracting a variety of computerised and internet marketing campaigns (Butcher 2008). The evidence for its efficacy in early dementia is thin, but when personalised to the individual, some benefits may be seen (Chapter 6). CR is based on developing individual goals that are meaningful to the person (Chapters 3 and

4) and that assist them to learn new ways of overcoming day-to-day memory related difficulties (Clare 2008). The Cochrane review on CST is positive, whilst that on CT and CR remains equivocal.

Equally familiar in many dementia care settings are activities such as reminiscence (Schweitzer 1998; Chapter 11), which uses autobiographical memories. These are often intact in early and moderate dementia. Reinforcing autobiographical memory in dementia through reminiscence may, like CST, CT and CR, be categorised as a cognition-orientated treatment. However in this book we have categorised reminiscence therapy as one that provides psychological and social support (Chapter 11) since:

- it is biased in favour of pleasant events which enhance feelings of well-being (Walker, Skowronski and Thompson 2003)

- it mostly depends on pleasurable social engagement with others (Bassett and Graham 2007)

- its expected outcomes, unlike CST, may have a greater impact on social interaction and quality of life than on cognition.

Although the 2005 Cochrane review did not find a strong evidence base for reminiscence, an eight-centre cluster randomised trial of couples group reminiscence (see also Chapter 11) by Woods and his colleagues is currently underway in the UK (www.controlled-trials.com/ISRCTN42430123, accessed 2 August 2008).

The family counselling programme of Mittelman and her colleagues (2003) in the USA, remains the most longstanding study of psychosocial intervention in dementia, with impressive outcomes reported (Mittelman *et al.* 2006). Extension of this trial in the Netherlands is currently underway (Joling *et al.* 2008) and other similar interventions directed at person–family dyads have also shown that it is possible to reduce distress in family carers through early psychosocial interventions and timely ongoing support (see the Seattle Protocols of Teri *et al.* 2005; Moniz-Cook *et al.* 2008a; Chapter 3). The UK BECCA randomised trial (Chapter 16) of a befriending service for family carers is also now complete. As noted in the opening paragraphs of this chapter, provision of individually tailored home-based programmes involving both the person with dementia and the family (Chapter 3) reflects the zeitgeist, that is, the state of the art in dementia care practice (Vernooij-Dassen and Moniz-Cook 2005). A recent example of this from the Netherlands provided in-home occupational therapy within a randomised trial, demonstrating positive outcomes on activities of daily living, skills, mood and quality of life in the person with dementia as well as an improved sense of competence in the primary family carer (Graff *et al.* 2006, 2007).

These approaches have much in common: they demonstrate a wide menu of interventions, where in many parts of Europe the skill base is already well developed. Organisations such as Alzheimer's Europe and INTERDEM (contact details at the end of chapter) offer opportunities for people with dementia, carers, practitioners, educators, researchers and policymakers to share skills and understandings. Strong traditions of psychology and a history of community-based practice are features of European health and social care practice that are sometimes overlooked. This is a workforce that has adapted to major changes in health and social care provision for people with dementia and has often stimulated such changes, notably the growing move from institutional care to community or home-based services.

At a time when services are resourced on the basis of rigorous consideration of treatments – such as in the case of pharmacological treatments in dementia care – it is possible that the next generation of practice developments may have to justify more explicitly the basis on which psychosocial interventions are delivered since competition for resources within dementia services will be fierce and common across Europe. The evidence base for early intervention services is small but growing, and likely to be of rising importance as resources lag ever far behind demand, and when more people with dementia or their representatives are, in parts of Europe, beginning themselves to purchase support services. One of the challenges will be to set out the costs as well as the benefits, to allow commissioners of dementia services to reach informed choices about what interventions can be afforded, since dementia services are often under-resourced (Macijauskiene 2007). Cost consequence studies are emerging for some psychosocial interventions such as group-based CST in the UK (Knapp *et al.* 2006) and in-home occupational therapy in the Netherlands (Graff *et al.* 2008). The growth in 'cash for care' services is remarkable across developed countries (see Breda *et al.* 2006) and practitioners offering psychosocial support will need to be more exact in estimations of staffing levels and optimum numbers for groups or activities in order that purchasing organisations, individuals and their proxies may properly evaluate the choices on offer.

Personalising psychosocial intervention

The chapters in this book outline the many psychosocial interventions and services that are available across Europe and beyond, and their limitations. What is special about this book is that the interventions are set in the evaluative tradition of dementia care and its aspirations to listen to the voices of people with dementia and their carers (see also Innes and McCabe 2007). Each chapter provides a conceptual basis for the intervention described, a summary of outcomes and a case illustration of how the intervention might be carried out in practice. Many of the interventions have arisen from randomised trials or from components of these, where the outcome measures applied in evaluation can also be used by the practitioner to measure outcomes in routine practice (Moniz-Cook *et al.* 2008b). The chapters are also strongly focused at proactive support to prevent further disability due to cognitive losses in older people. Therefore many of the interventions described are also applicable to people who have not yet developed a dementia but require a 'watching brief' over a number of years (Woods *et al.* 2003) or have mild cognitive impairments, since increasingly both pharmacological and psychosocial interventions are being considered as possible means of delaying the onset of dementia (Tuokko and Hultsch 2006).

There are three broad categories of early and timely psychosocial interventions described in this book that can be applied in practice: support at the time of diagnosis (Chapters 2–3); interventions to enhance cognition and memory (Chapters 4–8); and interventions to enhance psychological and social adjustment (Chapters 9–13). These can be used with people with dementia, or carers, or with both, although matching these to family circumstances in early dementia is not straightforward. For example, a recent systematic review of combined intervention programmes for people with dementia living at home and their families (Smits *et al.* 2007) concludes: 'Care professionals must define their programme goals and target groups before advising their clients' (p.1181).

Practice issues

In selecting psychosocial intervention(s) to assist the person with early dementia and/or the 'carer', practitioners need to consider a number of issues. First, the person's circumstances and wishes should be explored. An assessment framework for psychosocial intervention and rehabilitation in suspected or early dementia can be found in Moniz-Cook (2008). Selecting the relevant interventions will usually need a focused assessment combining personal profile, biography, interests, motivations and relationships for the person with suspected dementia as well as the close family or other supporters. Increasingly this may be done jointly or through self-assessment. This should enable the practitioner or team to work with the person in establishing what outcomes they wish to achieve and planning this support. Box 1.1, drawn from case studies in memory clinics and social care settings, illustrates some of the personal outcomes that people with early dementia may wish to achieve.

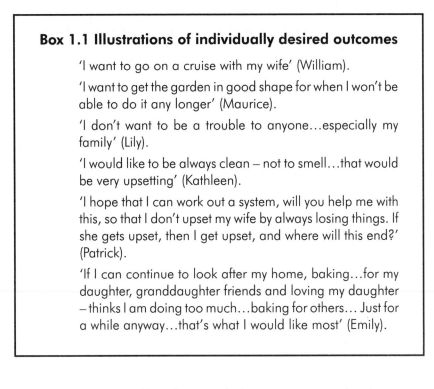

Box 1.1 Illustrations of individually desired outcomes

'I want to go on a cruise with my wife' (William).

'I want to get the garden in good shape for when I won't be able to do it any longer' (Maurice).

'I don't want to be a trouble to anyone...especially my family' (Lily).

'I would like to be always clean – not to smell...that would be very upsetting' (Kathleen).

'I hope that I can work out a system, will you help me with this, so that I don't upset my wife by always losing things. If she gets upset, then I get upset, and where will this end?' (Patrick).

'If I can continue to look after my home, baking...for my daughter, granddaughter friends and loving my daughter – thinks I am doing too much...baking for others... Just for a while anyway...that's what I would like most' (Emily).

Next the practitioner will need to consider how to arrange or plan the support offered, selected on the basis of possible options such as follows:

- Individually based support, often applied during visits to the family home or in outpatient clinics (as in Chapters 3, 4, 6, 8, 10, 11 and 15).

- Group-based support (as in Chapter 3, see post-diagnosis family workshops; Chapters 5, 7, 9 and 11 for couples group-based reminiscence; Chapters 12, 13 and 14), or the couples memory club intervention (Zarit *et al.* 2004).

- Inclusion of the family carer in the intervention with the person (Chapters 3, 4, 8, 11, 14, 15; Zarit *et al.* 2004); or support offered to the person or the carer in the absence of the other (for the person see Chapters 3, 4, 5, 6, 7, 8, 9, 10, 11 – where treatment is provided by supervised volunteers or therapists – and Chapter 12; for the carer see Chapters 13 and 16); or offering separate parallel group support to the person and the carer such as the meeting centres approach (Chapter 14) and the memory club, where opportunity to meet jointly as well as separately was offered (Zarit *et al.* 2004).

Group-based psychosocial intervention

Apart from Cognitive Stimulation Therapy and more recently Reminiscence Therapy, the evidence base for other types of group intervention is not strong. However the potential for this to develop in the future exists (Chapter 9; see Scott and Clare 2003 for a review). The decision to develop psychosocial group intervention programmes for people themselves (Chapter 9) or for family carers (Chapter 13) will remain a challenge for practitioners and service funders. In establishing the method, type and setting of group support, the practitioner will need to consider whether:

- by offering group-based support to the person or 'carer', where the latter may not actual perceive himself or herself as a 'carer', they might inadvertently undermine the natural established relationship(s) that have acted as the cornerstone for many successful psychosocial intervention programmes (see Chapter 3 and the Seattle Protocols of Teri *et al.* 2005)

- to offer gender-specific or culturally specific opportunities of group support (see Chapter 12; Lees 2006; Rainsford and Waring 2005)

- to develop groups for younger or older people with dementia or more widely (Burgess 2005; Randeria and Bond 2006)

- to offer joint person–carer groups, or whether these should be run in parallel but separately for person and carer (Rainsford and Waring 2005; Scott *et al.* 2002)

- the group should be time limited (Chapter 12) or provide long-term support (Randeria and Bond 2006); time-limited groups are often difficult to end (Bender 2006) probably due to new social relationships that develop)

- the group setting should be clinically based (Bender 2006; Rainsford and Waring 2005; Randeria and Bond 2006) or voluntary sector based (Burgess 2005; Pratt, Clare and Aggarwal 2005).

Decisions will depend on the function of the intervention and local resources, which will need to be discussed with the person and/or the 'carer'.

Targeting psychosocial interventions: towards unravelling complexity

To date research in dementia care has little systematic advice to offer the practitioner in how to select psychosocial intervention(s). Furthermore, it is not known whether group-based support is more effective than individualised home-based support in maintaining quality of life by delaying distress and associated burden, for both the person with dementia and the family. In this final section we will use the current and emerging evidence base outlined above (and in the first three parts of this book), to suggest stepped principles for the selection of psychosocial intervention in early dementia.

For detailed background in assessment for psychosocial intervention in early dementia, the reader is referred to Moniz-Cook (2008), which draws from knowledge and experience of older people and their families at the point of recognition and includes the individual and sometimes distinct psychological strengths and needs of both. For example, where an intervention is offered too early, this may exacerbate support needs; or in-home individualised early intervention increased carer anxiety over the three months of one intervention, but when pleasurable activity was added, longer term distress and burden were less (Chapter 3).

As a starting point to our framework for selecting evidence-based interventions in early dementia, we return to our previous discussion on the role of attitudes – sometimes underpinned by stigma – in the development and uptake of psychosocial services in early dementia. To counteract this we suggest that interventions should be guided by social models of disability, with the disease model restricted to descriptions of specific neurological impairments (Chapter 3). This perspective allows the practitioner to intervene to promote health and well-being and thus prevent or minimise the extra disability of distress and reduced mood in older people with suspected dementia and their families. To achieve this by personalising intervention to need and context, we suggest the following stepped care framework for psychosocial interventions in early dementia:

- *Step 1 interventions* should use the time of diagnosis as an opportunity to address stigmatised attitudes and provide methods of promoting health and well-being in early dementia (Chapters 2, 3). Diagnostic disclosure programmes are developing (Derksen *et al.* 2006) as are methods to address fears by focusing on strengths and abilities (Chapter 3). A general principle would be: to promote in-home cognitive rehabilitation or training (Chapters 3, 4, 6) or provide technologies (Chapter 8) to enhance a sense of control over memory; to reinforce usual family and social support networks and associated activities (Chapter 3, 16); to involve, where possible, both the person and the family 'carer'. Reminiscence activity (Chapter 11) can also be another means of strengthening family relationships.

- *Step 2 interventions* include evidence-based groups that are prophylactic in nature in that they do not target those that are already distressed. They will best suit people with early dementia and their families who do not have adequate opportunity for mental stimulation and social activity and valued friendships in their natural environment. Evidence-based groups include Cognitive Stimulation Therapy (Chapters 5, 6, 7) and Reminiscence Therapy (Chapter 11).

- *Step 3 interventions* are those described under the *social inclusion* umbrella, where a strong focus on opportunity for social engagement and voluntary sector support in communities is the norm. These interventions – such as the 'Alzheimer's Café' (Campus 2005; Miesen and Blom 2001) – tend not to be time limited and offer the opportunity for the shared experience of having dementia to reinforce social identity. We suggest that some of the difficulties encountered when time-limited groups have to end their programmes, including those in Step 2, may be overcome by having in place a regular (perhaps monthly) Alzheimer's Café to allow people and their families to maintain their social contact and support of each other. In some early dementia care services, Alzheimer's Cafés appear to act as the only post-diagnosis ongoing support service alternative to anti-dementia drug treatment (Thompson 2006, p.295). Alternatively, where social relationships have been undermined by the effects of dementia, as is common in younger people who develop dementia, or people have become socially isolated for some other reason and Step 1 intervention is not possible, structured support to engage in services for people with dementia such as the Talking About Memory Coffee Club (Pratt *et al.* 2005) or internet-based social support may be considered.

- *Step 4 interventions* include individual and group therapy for the person with dementia who may be distressed and require support to adjust to the knowledge of having dementia or to recover their sense of self-identity (Chapters 9, 10; see Moniz-Cook 2008 for examples of psychological treatments for distress in early dementia). This category may also include:

o group support to enhance competence and/or social support or pleasure for the person with dementia or the 'carer' (Chapters 11, 12, 13)

o individual social support for either the person or the 'carer' through befriending schemes (Nicholson 2005; Chapter 16)

o personal counselling, treatment and supportive intervention for the 'carer', where ongoing service support systems (Part IV) become important in sustaining positive outcomes over time.

Table 1.2 summarises guidance for assisting practitioners to make informed choices on what interventions might be appropriate to offer people with early dementia and families, taking into account their personal and in some cases differing needs.

Conclusion

The four parts of this book are unified by their focus on the requirement that interventions and services should be personalised to outcomes, need and context. While we accept the importance of models of disability and organisational systems, the authors frequently return to emotions, worries and concerns of people and their families, probably because most are research practitioners who are in frequent contact with people with dementia and their supporters. Organisational and service contexts will remain important, as is highlighted by the multidisciplinary background of chapter contributors who, as can be seen in Part IV of this book, often work across settings and boundaries. Finally, our pan-European theme, wherein practitioners and researchers have accepted the challenge to describe their service and activities to readers who may be unfamiliar with particular national contexts, has the potential for raising the quality of responses to dementia across countries. As in the case of the psychosocial interventions of Mary Mittelman from New York, now being tested in the Netherlands, chapter contents may be drawn upon and transferred to other countries across Europe and beyond. This inter-nation communication enabled the genesis of this book, when a multiprofessional group of individuals discovered that there was more that united than divided them in their aspirations to support people with early dementia and their families. These conversations led to a thriving multiprofessional European research practice network INTERDEM, which continues to inspire, communicate and

Table 1.2 Guidelines for choosing psychosocial intervention

BOOK SECTION	AIM	TASKS OF INTERVENTION	GUIDELINES
Support around diagnosis	Neutralise stigma	To separate 'brain from mind'	Provide person and the carer with verbal and written information on retained aspects of cognition, how areas of deficit might impact on everyday living and what they might do to overcome the subtle changes in function that they experience (Chapter 3).
		To address myths /rehabilitative nihilism	Address issues of uncertainty, possible concerns of family members and/or health and social care professionals surrounding 'how to tell' a diagnosis. Discussion should focus on understanding the meaning of dementia for the person and for family members or other supporters and providing them with information, options and avenues to overcome fear or nihilistic views about maintaining well-being and quality of life (Chapter 2; see also Moniz-Cook 2008). Consider opportunities for psychosocial intervention (Chapter 2).
			Use the discussion to negotiate interventions (from the tool kit in Sections 2–4) that might minimise the risks of anxiety, depression, disability or distress for both the person and the primary supporting family member. Consider with caution wheter attending a 'class' is perceived as a meaningful activity (see below) and also the appropriateness of out-of-home structured group activity such as cognitive stimulation (Chapter 7), therapy (Chapters 9, 10, 12, 13), unless the person or carer is unduly distressed.
Cognition-focused intervention	Individualis-ing the intervention to prevent 'excess disability'	To enhance control and minimise worry in the person with dementia	Where a high need for cognitive control and a belief in the 'use it or lose it' hypothesis is observed, consider establishing cognition maintaining strategies (Chapter 3), cognitive rehabilitation or training (Chapters 4, 6), or technology if available (Chapter 8) to address meaningful personal rehabilitative goals or in-home cognitive stimulation (Onder et al. 2005).
			Where previous participation in adult education classes or activity in group-based facilities is noted and a person is not shy and therefore likely with encouragement to engage in group activity, consider offering structured time-limited group cognitive stimulation (Chapters 5, 7).
			Discuss with person and carer the pros and cons of introducing for the first time crosswords or other mental activity and whether these are of value or provide pleasure.
Psychological and social support		To support the distressed carer	Generally involving the carer is beneficial to both (Chapters 3, 4 and see Onder et al. 2005). Where families are distressed at subtle changes in their relative, avoid their initial involvement in cognition-orientated programmes and consider in-home or group-based reminiscence (Chapter 11).
		To support the distressed person and/or carer	Offer carer counselling or support (Chapters 13, 16); or take a co-ordinated Meeting Centre approach (Chapter 14) where the person may participate in group cognitive stimulation or in developing personal support outside the family (Chapters 5, 7, 12) whilst the relative receives group-based support (Chapter 13).

Managing distress	To provide psychosocial treatment to minimise/reduce distress	Where anxiety and distress about 'losing their mind' is noted, consider individual therapy (Chapter 10), group therapy (Chapter 9) or supported behavioural activation to prevent depression (Chapter 3).
		If anxiety is not high but subtle social withdrawal from pleasurable social contacts or activities is a risk, consider individual support to re-engage in pleasurable activity through cognitive rehabilitation (Chapter 4) or behavioural activation (Chapter 3) or through provision of new opportunities for pleasurable group resocialisation (Chapter 12).
		For younger people with dementia avoid premature reminiscence activity. Consider psychotherapy (Chapters 9, 10), group support (Chapter 12) or individual counselling (see Moniz-Cook 2008).
	Sustaining strong family relationships	Consider family-supported reminiscence as a tool for identify maintenance activity and also for engaging in pleasurable activity (Chapter 11).
Establishing supportive services	Maintaining the effects of early intervention	Preventing burden and maintaining long-term quality of life	Consider in most cases support for both parts of the person–carer dyad (Chapters 14, 15) or the carer alone (Chapters 13, 16).
		Where there are strong fears of dementia or evidence of 'protective care-giving' (Gillies 1995) consider offering couples or family-based workshops (Chapter 3) and reminiscence (Chapter 11).

develop new psychosocial research in dementia care. Our aspiration is that the contents of this book will further extend these conversations and that this book will offer something for those who echo the call of practitioners and people with early dementia across Europe, epitomised by a recent call from France: 'We need multi-component interventions to effectively slow down the disablement process' (Jacques Touchon, neurologist, in interview with Dorenlot, 2007, p.11).

Note

1　　In this chapter families, spouses, partners and relatives have sometimes been referred to as 'carers' with deliberate quotation marks, since at recognition/diagnosis and the years that can precede this neither they nor the person with suspected dementia may perceive them as a carer. In subsequent chapters we have, for ease, used the term carer without parentheses.

References

Bamford, C., Lamont, S., Eccles, M., Robinson, L., May, C. and Bond, J. (2004) 'Disclosing a diagnosis of dementia: a systematic review.' *International Journal of Geriatric Psychiatry 19*, 151–169.

Bassett, R. and Graham, J.E. (2007) 'Memorabilities: enduring relationships, memories and abilities in dementia.' *Ageing and Society 27*, 533–554.

Beavis, D. (2007) 'The Alzheimer's Medication Service: Developing an Early Intervention Service in a Rural Community.' In J. Keady, C. Clarke and S. Page (eds) *Partnerships in Community Mental Health Nursing and Dementia Care: Practice Perspectives.* Maidenhead: Open University Press.

Benbow, S. and Reynolds, D. (2000) 'Challenging the stigma of Alzheimer's disease.' *Hospital Medicine 61*, 174–177.

Bender, M. (2006) 'The Wadebridge Memory Bank Group and beyond.' *PSIGE – Psychology Specialists Promoting Psychological Wellbeing in Late Life – Newsletter 95*, 28–33.

Bird, M. (2000) 'Psychosocial Rehabilitation for Problems arising from Cognitive Deficits in Dementia.' In R.D. Hill, L. Backman and A.S. Neely (eds) *Cognitive Rehabilitation in Old Age.* Oxford: Oxford University Press.

Breda, J., Schoenmaekers, D., Van Landeghem, C., Claessens, D. and Geerts, J. (2006) 'When Informal Care becomes a Paid Job: The Case of Personal Assistance Budgets in Flanders.' In C. Glendinning and P. Kemp (eds) *Cash and Care: Policy Challenges in the Welfare State.* Bristol: The Policy Press.

Brodaty, H., Green, A. and Koschera, A. (2003) 'Meta-analysis of psychosocial interventions for caregivers of people with dementia.' *Journal of the American Geriatrics Society 51*, 657–664.

Bryden-Boden, C. (2002) 'A person-centred approach to counselling, psychotherapy and rehabilitation of people with dementia in the early stages.' *Dementia 1*, 141–156.

Burgener, S.C. and Berger, B. (2008) 'Measuring perceived stigma in persons with progressive neurological disease: Alzheimer's dementia and Parkinson's disease.' *Dementia 7*, 31–53.

Buntinx, F., De Lepeleire, J., Fontaine, O. and Ylieff M. (2002) *Qualidem Final Report 1999–2002, version 1.1*, Qualidem: Leuven/Liège.

Burgess, R. (2005) 'The Deep Thinkers Group.' *Journal of Dementia Care 13*, 22–25.

Butcher, J. (2008) 'Mind games: do they work?' *British Medical Journal 336*, 246–248.

Cameron, C. and Moss, P. (2007) *Carework in Europe.* London: Routledge.

Camp, C.J., Bird, M. and Cherry, K.E. (2000) 'Retrieval Strategies as a Rehabilitation Aid for Cognitive Loss in Pathological Aging.' In R.D. Hill, L. Backman and A.S. Neely (eds) *Cognitive Rehabilitation in Old Age.* Oxford: Oxford University Press.

Campus, J. (2005) 'The Kingston Dementia Café: the benefits of establishing an Alzheimer's café for carers and people with dementia.' *Dementia 4*, 588–591.

Clare, L. (2008) *Neuropsychological Rehabilitation and People with Dementia.* Hove: Psychology Press.

Clare, L. and Woods, R.T. (eds) (2001) *Cognitive Rehabilitation in Dementia.* Hove: Psychology Press.

Clare, L., Rowlands, J. and Quin, R. (2008) 'Collective strength: the impact of developing a shared social identity in early-stage dementia.' *Dementia 7*, 9–30.

de Boer, M.E., Hertogh, C.M.P., Dröes, R., Ripinhagen, I.I., Jonker, C. and Eefsting, J.A. (2007) 'Suffering from dementia – the patient's perspective; a review of the literature.' *International Psychogeriatrics 19*, 1021–1039.

Derksen, E., Vernooij-Dassen, M., Scheltens, P. and Olde Rikkert, M. (2006) 'A model for disclosure of the diagnosis of dementia.' *Dementia 5*, 462–468.

Di Carlo, A., Baldereschi, M., S. *et al.* for the Ilsa Group (The Italian Longitudinal Study on Aging Working Group) (2002). 'Incidence of dementia, Alzheimer's disease and vascular dementia in Italy.' *Journal of the American Geriatrics Society 50*, 41–48.

Friedell, M. and Bryden-Boden, C. (2002) 'Guest editorial: a word from two turtles.' *Dementia 1*, 131–133.

Gillies, B. (1995) 'The subjective experience of dementia – a qualitative analysis of interviews with dementia suffers and their carers and the implications for service provision.' PhD thesis, University of Dundee, UK.

Goffman, G.E. (1963) *Stigma: Notes on the Management of Spoiled Identity*. New York, NY: Prentice Hall.

Graff, M.J.L., Vernooij-Dassen, M., Thijssen, M., Dekker, J., Hoefnagels, W.H.L. and Olde Rikkert, M.G.M. (2006) 'Community based occupational therapy for patients with dementia and their caregivers: randomised controlled trial.' *British Medical Journal 333*, 1196–2002.

Graff, M.J.L., Vernooij-Dassen, M., Thijssen, M., Dekker, J., Hoefnagels, W.H.L. and Olde Rikkert, M.G.M. (2007) 'Effects of community occupational therapy on quality of life, mood, and health status in dementia patients and their caregivers: a randomized controlled trial.' *Journals of Gerontology Series A: Biological Sciences; Medical Sciences 62*, 1002–1009.

Graff, M.J.L., Adang E.M.M., Vernooij-Dassen, M.J.M., Jönsson, J.L., *et al.* (2008) 'Community occupational therapy for older patients with dementia and their care givers: cost effectiveness study.' *British Medical Journal 336*, 134–138.

Heller, T. and Heller, L. (2003) Editorial. 'First among equals? Does drug treatment claim more than its fair share of resources?' *Dementia 2*, 7–19.

Iliffe, S. and Manthorpe, J. (2004) Editorial. 'The hazards of early recognition of dementia: a risk assessment.' *Aging and Mental Health 8*, 99–105.

Iliffe, S., De Lepeleire, J., van Hout, H., Kenny, G., Lewis A., Vernooij-Dassen, M. and the DIADEM group (2005) 'Understanding obstacles to the recognition of and response to dementia in different European countries: a modified focus group approach using multinational, multi-disciplinary expert groups.' *Aging and Mental Health 9*, 1–6.

Ilsa Group (The Longitudinal Study on Aging Working Group) (1997) 'Prevalence of Chronic diseases in older Italians: comparing self-reported and clinical diagnoses.' *International Journal of Epidemiology 26*, 995–1002.

Innes, A. and McCabe, L. (eds) (2007) *Evaluation in Dementia Care*. London: Jessica Kingsley Publishers.

Jansen, A.P., van Hout, H.P., van Marwijk, H.W., Nijpels, G., *et al.* (2005) 'Cost-effectiveness of case-management by district nurses among primary informal caregivers of older adults with dementia symptoms and the older adults who receive informal care: design of a randomized controlled trial.' PMID: 16343336. *BMC Public Health 12*, 5, 133.

Joling, K.J., van Hout, H.P., Scheltens, P., Vernooij-Dassen, M. *et al.* (2008) 'Cost-effectiveness of family meetings on indicated prevention of anxiety and depressive symptoms and disorders of primary family caregivers of patients with dementia: design of a randomized controlled trial.' PMID: 18208607. *BMC Geriatrics 8*, 1, 2.

Katsuno, T (2005) 'Dementia from the inside: how people with early-stage dementia evaluate their quality of life.' *Ageing and Society 25*, 197–214.

Keady, J., Clarke, C. and Page, S. (eds) (2007) *Partnerships in Community Mental Health Nursing and Dementia Care: Practice Perspectives*. Maidenhead: Open University Press.

Keogh, F. and Roche, A. (1996) *Mental disorders in older Irish People*. National Council for the Elderly, Dublin, Report No.45.

Knapp, M., Thorgrimsen, L., Patel, A., Spector, A. *et al.* (2006) 'Cognitive Stimulation Therapy for dementia: is it cost effective?' *British Journal of Psychiatry 188*, 574–580.

Launer, L.J., Anderson, K., Dewey, M.E., Letemeur, L., Ott, A., Amadueci, L.A. *et al. 'Rates and risk factors for dementia and Alzheimer's disease: results from EURODEM pooled analyses. EURODEM Incidence Research Group and Work Groups. European Syudies of Dementia. Neurology 52*, 1, 78–84.

Lees, K. (2006) 'Gentlemen who lunch: developing self-help groups for people with early diagnosis of dementia.' *PSIGE – Psychology Specialists Promoting Psychological Wellbeing in Late Life – Newsletter 96*, 33–37.

Lobo, A., Saz, P., Marcos, G., Dia, J.L., de la Ca'mara, C. (1995) 'The Prevalence of Dementia and Depression in the Elderly Community in a South European Population: The Zaragoza study.' Arch Gen Psychiatry 52: 497–506.

Macijauskiene, J. (2007) 'Evaluation of dementia care in resource-scarce settings.' In A. Innes and L. McCabe (eds) *Evaluation in Dementia Care*. London: Jessica Kingsley Publishers.

Miesen, B.M.L. and Blom, M. (2001) *The Alzheimer Café: A Guideline Manual for Setting One Up*. Translated and adapted from the Dutch Alzheimer's Society document by G.M.M. Jones. Available at www.alzheimercafeuk.co.uk, accessed 5 August 2008.

Mittelman, M.S., Epstein, C. and Pierzchala, A. (2003) *Counseling the Alzheimer's Caregiver: A Resource for Health Care Professionals*. Chicago: American Medical Association Press.

Mittelman, M.S., William, P.H., Haley, E., Clay, O. and Roth, D. (2006) 'Improving caregiver well-being delays nursing home placement of patients with Alzheimer disease.' *Neurology 67*, 1592–1599.

Moise, P., Schwarzinger, M., Myung-Yong, U. and the Dementia Expert Group. (2004) *Dementia Care in 9 OECD countries: A Comparative Analysis*. Paris: OECD Health Working Papers 13.

Moniz-Cook, E. (2006) Editorial: 'Cognitive stimulation in dementia.' *Aging and Mental Health 10*, 207–210.

Moniz-Cook, E.D. (2008) 'Assessment and Psychosocial Intervention for Older People with Suspected Dementia: A Memory Clinic Perspective.' In K. Laidlaw and B. Knight (eds) *Handbook of Emotional Disorders in Late Life: Assessment and Treatment*. Oxford: Oxford University Press.

Moniz-Cook, E.D., Manthorpe, J., Carr, I., Gibson, G. and Vernooij-Dassen, M. (2006) 'Facing the future: a qualitative study of older people referred to a memory clinic prior to assessment and diagnosis.' *Dementia 5*, 375–395.

Moniz-Cook, E.D., Elston, C., Gardiner, E., Agar, S., *et al.* (2008a) 'Can training community mental health nurses to support family carers reduce behavioural problems in dementia? An exploratory pragmatic randomised controlled trial.' *International Journal of Geriatric Psychiatry 23*, 185–191.

Moniz-Cook, E., Vernooij-Dassen, M., Woods, R., Verhey, F., *et al.* (2008b) 'A European consensus on outcome measures for psychosocial intervention research in dementia care.' *Aging and Mental Health 12*, 3–19.

National Institute of Health and Clinical Excellence (NICE) and Social Care Institute for Excellence (SCIE) (2006) *Dementia: Supporting People with Dementia and their Carers*. Clinical Guideline 42. London: NICE.

Nicholson, L. (2005) 'The value of enjoying life side by side: a befriending scheme in Nottinghamshire, UK.' *Journal of Dementia Care 13*, 3, 14–16.

Onder, G., Zanetti, O., Giacobini, E., Frisoni, G., *et al.* (2005) 'Reality orientation therapy combined with cholinesterase inhibitors in Alzheimer's disease: randomised controlled trial.' *British Journal of Psychiatry 187*, 450–455.

Ott, A., Breteler, M.M.B., Harskamp van, F., Claus, J.J., Cammen van der T.J.M., Grobbee, D.E., Hofman, A. (1995) 'Prevalence of Alzheimer's disease and vascular dementia: association with education. The Rotterdam study. *British Medical Journal 310*, 970–97.

Page, S. (2007) 'Nurse Prescribing and the CMHN: Assuming New Responsibilities in Dementia Treatment.' In J. Keady, C. Clarke and S. Page (eds) *Partnerships in Community Mental Health Nursing and Dementia Care: Practice Perspectives*. Maidenhead: Open University Press.

Parahoo, K., Campbell, A. and Scoltock, C. (2002) 'An evaluation of a domiciliary respite service for younger people with dementia.' *Journal of Evaluation in Clinical Practice 8*, 4, 377–385.

Pratt, R., Clare, L. and Aggarwal, N. (2005) 'The talking about memory group: a new model for support for people with early-stage dementia and their families.' *Dementia 4*, 143–148.

Rainsford, C. and Waring, J. (2005) 'Support groups offer a lifeline.' *Journal of Dementia Care 13*, 3, 13–14.

Ramaroson, H., Helmer, C., Baberger-Gateau, P., Letenneur, L., Dartigues, J-F. (2003) 'Prevalence of dementia and Alzheimer's disease among subjects aged 75 years or over: updated results of PAQUID cohort.' *Revue Neurologique 159*, 4, 405–411.

Randeria, L. and Bond, J. (2006) 'The Phoenix Group – living again after a diagnosis of dementia.' *PSIGE – Psychology Specialists Promoting Psychological Wellbeing in Late Life – Newsletter 93*, 26–29.

Ruitenberg, A., Ott, A., Swieten, van J.C., Hofman, A., Breteler, M.M.B., (2001) 'Incidence of dementia: does gender make a difference?' *Neurobiological Aging 22*, 575–580.

Schweitzer, P. (ed.) (1998) *Reminiscence in Dementia Care*. London: Age Exchange.

Scott, J. and Clare, L. (2003) 'Do people with dementia benefit from psychological interventions offered on a group basis?' *Clinical Psychology and Psychotherapy 10*, 186–196.

Scott, J., Clare, L., Charlesworth, G. and Luckie, M. (2002) 'Parallel groups for people with dementia and their partners.' *PSIGE – Psychology Specialists Promoting Psychological Wellbeing in Late Life – Newsletter, 80*, 18–22.

Scottish Intercollegiate Guidelines Network (SIGN) (2006) *Management of Patients with Dementia: A National Clinical Guideline*. Edinburgh: SIGN.

Smits, C.H.M., de Lange, J., Dröes, R.M., Meiland, F., Vernooij-Dassen, M. and Pot, A.M. (2007) 'Effects of combined intervention programmes for people with dementia living at home and their caregivers: a systematic review.' *International Journal of Geriatric Psychiatry 22*, 1181–1193.

Stern, Y. (ed.) (2007) *Cognitive Reserve: Theory and Applications*. New York, NY: Taylor and Francis.

Teri, L., McCurry, S.M., Logsdon, R. and Gibbons, L.E. (2005) 'Training community consultants to help family members improve dementia care.' *Gerontologist 45*, 802–811.

Thompson, A. (2006) 'Qualitative Evaluation of an Alzheimer café as an Ongoing Support Group Intervention.' In B.M.L. Miesen and G.M.M Jones (eds) *Care-giving in Dementia: Research and Applications*, Vol. 4. London and New York, NY: Routledge.

Touchon, J. and Dorenlot, P. (2007) 'We need multi-component interventions to effectively slow down the disablement process.' In P. Dorenlot and M. Frémontier (eds) *Non-Pharmacological Interventions in Dementia*. Paris: Les Cahiers de la Fondation Médéric Alzheimer, 3, 10–13.

Tuokko, H.A. and Hultsch, D.F. (2006) *Mild Cognitive Impairment: International Perspectives*. New York, NY: Taylor and Francis.

Vernooij-Dassen, M. and Moniz-Cook, E. (2005) 'Improving the quality of in home interventions in dementia care.' *Dementia 4*, 165–169.

Vernooij-Dassen, M., Moniz-Cook, E., Woods, R., De Lepeleire, J., *et al.* (2005) 'Factors affecting timely recognition and diagnosis of dementia across Europe: from awareness to stigma.' *International Journal of Geriatric Psychiatry 20*, 377–386.

Vilalta-Franch, J., Lopez-Pousa, S., Llinas-Regla, J. (2000) 'La prevalencia de demencias en un area rural. Un estudio en Gerona.' Revue Neurologique 11, 1026-1032.

Walker, W.R., Skowronski, J.J. and Thompson, C.P. (2003) 'Life is pleasant – and memory helps to keep it that way!' *Review of General Psychology 7*, 203–210.

Warner, M., Furnish, S., Longley, M. and Lawlor, B. (eds) (2002) *Alzheimer's Disease: Policy and Practice across Europe*. Oxford: Radcliffe Medical Press.

Wind, A., Gussekloo, J., Vernooij-Dassen, M., Bouma, M., Boomsma, L.J. and Boukes, F.S. (2003) 'NHG-Standaard Dementie (tweede herziening) Dutch Dementia Guidelines' (second revision). *Huisarts Wet 46*, 754–766.

Woods, B. (2003) 'Evidence-based practice in psychosocial intervention in early dementia: how can it be achieved?' *Aging and Mental Health 7*, 5–6.

Woods, R.T., Moniz-Cook, E.D., Iliffe, S., Campion, P., *et al.* (2003) 'Dementia: issues in early recognition and intervention in primary care.' *Journal of the Royal College of Medicine 96*, 320–324.

Ylieff, M., Fontaine, O., De Lepeleire, J., and Buntinx, F. (2002) Qualidem Final Report 1999–2002: Qualidem: Liège/Leuven.

Zarit, S.H, Femia, E.E., Watson, J., Rice-Oeschger, L. and Kakos, B. (2004) 'Memory club: a group intervention for people with early stage dementia and their care partners.' *The Gerontologist 44*, 262–269.

Websites

Alzheimer's Disease International. www.alz.co.uk (accessed 5 August 2008)

Alzheimers Europe. www.alzheimers-europe.org (accessed 5 August 2008)

Cognitive stimulation. www.cstdementia.com/index.php (accessed 5 August 2008)

DASNI – the international internet-based Dementia Advocacy and Support Network. www.dasninternational.org (accessed 5 August 2008)

INTERDEM. http://interdem.alzheimer-europe.org (accessed 5 August 2008)

REMCARE. www.controlled-trials.com/ISRCTN42430123 (accessed 5 August 2008)

Table 1.1. www.who.int/mental_health (accessed 5 August 2008)

Topic Dementia and Cognitive Improvement. www.mrw.interscience.wiley.com/cochrane

Related Cochrane protocols and reviews

Clare, L., Woods, R.T., Moniz-Cook, E.D., Orrell, M. and Spector, A. (2003) 'Cognitive rehabilitation and cognitive training interventions targeting memory functioning in early stage Alzheimer's disease and vascular dementia (review).' In *The Cochrane Library Database of Systematic Reviews*, Issue 4. Chichester: Wiley.

Martin, M., Clare, L. Altgassen, M. and Cameron, M. (2006) 'Cognition-based interventions for older people and people with mild cognitive impairment. (protocol.)' In *The Cochrane Library Database of Systematic Reviews*, Issue 4. Chichester: Wiley.

Vernooij-Dassen, M. and Downs, M. (2005) 'Cognitive and behavioural interventions for carers of people with dementia (protocol).' In *The Cochrane Library Database of Systematic Reviews*, Issue 2. Chichester: Wiley.

Woods, B., Spector, A., Jones, C., Orrell, M. and Davies, S. (2005) 'Reminiscence therapy for people with dementia. (review).' In *The Cochrane Library Database of Systematic Reviews*, Issue 2. Chichester: Wiley.

Woods, B., Spector, A., Prendergast, L. and Orrell, M. (2005) 'Cognitive stimulation to improve cognitive functioning in people with dementia (protocol).' In *The Cochrane Library Database of Systematic Reviews*, Issue 4. Chichester: Wiley.

Resources and further reading

Bender, M. (2004) *Therapeutic Groupwork for People with Cognitive Losses: Working with People with Dementia.* Milton Keynes: Speechmark.

Bender, M., Bauchham, P. and Norris, A. (1999) *The Therapeutic Purposes of Reminiscence.* London: Sage.

Spector, A., Thorgrimsen, L., Woods, B. and Orrell, M. (2006) *Making a Difference: An Evidence-based Group Programme to offer Cognitive Stimulation Therapy (CST) to People with Dementia. The Manual for Group Leaders.* London: Hawker Publications.

Woods, R.T. and Clare, L. (2006) 'Cognition-based Therapies and Mild Cognitive Impairment.' In H.A. Tuokko and D.F Hultsch (eds) *Mild Cognitive Impairment: International Perspectives.* New York, NY: Taylor and Francis.

Woods, R.T. and Clare, L. (2008) 'Psychological Intervention and Dementia.' In R.T. Woods and L. Clare (eds) *Handbook of the Clinical Psychology of Ageing*, 2nd edn. Chichester: Wiley.

PART I

Support at the Time of Diagnosis

Chapter 2

What Do We Tell People with Dementia about Their Diagnosis and How Do We Tell Them?

Hilary J. Husband

Overview

Giving someone the news that they have dementia is understandably something that many professionals find difficult to do. The person may feel a sense of loss, of stigmatism, and of hopelessness as a result. Coupled with this is the complication that a definite diagnosis may be problematic for some individuals. It is a recent development that health care professionals now consider telling the person their diagnosis, and this chapter explores issues facing both professionals and carers. A case example is also described, which highlights the advantages of early disclosure.

> It feels as though my brain is being taken away, bit by bit. I get scared, and then I remember it's this Alzheimer's disease. (Kathryn, a 72-year-old woman with dementia)

Dementia is one of the disorders that people most dread, especially the old, who are at most risk of its development. It is a disorder that carries a social stigma, is progressive and is associated with increasing dependency on others. It is also a disorder in which an individual's very sense of their self can be gradually eroded. It is perhaps not surprising that health professionals, who are only too aware of the losses inherent in dementia, find it difficult to talk to people about the experience.

The person-centred approach to dementia care identifies the 'malignant social psychology' that attaches itself to the condition. This includes attitudes from caregivers that serve to disempower the person with dementia and to undermine their sense of personhood (e.g. Kitwood 1997). This process can start very early in the course of dementia if it is assumed that people cannot be told what is causing the problems they have with their memory and other cognitive functions. If no one explains what is happening to them, they cannot express their wishes about their care and cannot be helped to understand their own situation.

How has the situation changed?

> We used to sweep all that sort of thing, mental problems and that, under the carpet, but not now. Now you talk about it. (Ron, a 78-year-old man who cares for his wife who has dementia)

The question of whether to tell people with dementia about their diagnosis has only recently been considered by health professionals in the UK. Whilst we accept that carers should be as fully informed as possible about dementia, there is considerably less certainty about informing people with dementia themselves. The issue has become more pressing as people are presenting earlier to services, when cognition is less impaired and it is easier to engage in discussion of diagnostic issues. The improved public awareness of dementia is a major factor in earlier presentation. Expectations of information giving from health professionals may also have changed in favour of greater openness.

The situation with dementia parallels that of cancer diagnoses in the 1960s, when a study found that 90 per cent of physicians did not normally inform patients they had cancer. It was felt the diagnosis was too hopeless and distressing, which would result in patients 'giving up' and perhaps becoming suicidal (Oken 1961). By 1979 the situation had reversed, with over 90 per cent of physicians being in favour of telling the patient the diagnosis whenever possible (Novak *et al.* 1979). Perhaps, as a result, the considerable stigma once surrounding cancer has now almost disappeared. It is noted by Novak *et al.* that most reluctance to disclose was expressed where the patient was old, of lower educational level and considered to have low intellectual ability. This suggests interesting parallels with people with dementia, who are mainly old, who as a cohort may have had little educational opportunity and whose cognitive impairments can make them appear less able.

There are, of course, important ethical principles to consider including the patient's 'right to know' as well as that of withholding information to prevent harm (Gillon 1985). Health professionals and carers have reasonable concerns that learning a diagnosis may lead to distress, stigmatisation and depression, although there is little empirical evidence to support this view (Meyers 1997). In terms of not telling the diagnosis the following arguments need to be considered:

- The diagnosis may be wrong.

- The diagnosis may be uncertain.

- There may be no treatment to offer.

- The individual may be unable to understand or remember information.

- The individual may refuse to accept, or deny the diagnosis.

- The diagnosis may be too distressing, leading to depressive withdrawal or suicide risk.

There are also good reasons why people should be told their diagnosis:

- They may ask to be told.

- They may already suspect the diagnosis.

- They can be consulted about decisions relating to their care.

- They have a framework for understanding their problems.

- They can talk openly to carers so secrecy and exclusion are avoided.

- They may wish to make a will, an advance decision or address family issues whilst still able to do so.

How many people with dementia are told their diagnosis?

> Mum kept crying and asking what was wrong with her. The nurse said just to tell her she had a memory problem. (Karen, a 37-year-old woman whose mother has dementia)

It is difficult to obtain a valid estimate of the proportion of people with dementia who learn their diagnosis. Most studies are surveys relying on self-report of attitudes and behaviour. People answering questionnaires may have poor recall of events, may underestimate or overestimate aspects of their behaviour, or may give the response they feel is most socially desirable. It would be very difficult to observe directly what people said about dementia to people with the condition, as the very act of being observed can alter behaviour. The population of people with dementia is diverse, and little is known of the characteristics of those who are told their diagnosis in comparison to those who are not.

A number of studies in the 1990s attempted to examine the question of just how often health professionals did disclose a dementia diagnosis. A study of consultant old age psychiatrists found that nearly half, 48 per cent, said they would tell somebody with mild dementia, in about 80 per cent of cases. Where dementia was more severe, only 10 per cent would consider telling the diagnosis. This suggests that less than half of those with mild dementia learn their diagnosis from a consultant. All of the respondents in this study reported that they told the carers of the diagnosis at all times (Rice and Warner 1994). A study of GPs found that 5 per cent reported they always told people their diagnosis, 34 per cent often told the diagnosis and 42 per cent occasionally told the diagnosis, again suggesting diagnosis is often withheld (Vassilas 1999).

A study of 20 memory clinics, where they specialise in diagnosing dementia, found that only 45 per cent of clinics reported that they discussed diagnosis with patients and only 37.5 per cent had any written guidelines on the issue (Gilliard and Gwilliam 1996). Given that memory clinics are centres of expertise, the neglect of disclosure issues is surprising.

It is not always a health professional who tells the person with dementia their diagnosis. A study of 42 carers found that in only two cases had a health professional told the person with dementia the diagnosis. A further nine carers (21.4%) had imparted the diagnosis themselves but only four carers (9.5%) had received any guidance or advice from a health professional on this issue (Husband 1996). A further study of carers comparing disclosure in early and late onset dementia found 48 per cent of people with dementia overall were told their diagnosis. There was no overall difference in rates of disclosure for younger and older people with dementia, but health professionals were significantly more likely to tell younger people than older people (Heal and Husband 1998).

Why do carers choose to tell or not to tell?

> How can you tell him something like that? He was always such a proud man, it's like telling him he's on the scrap heap, it would break him completely. (Joan, a 70-year-old woman caring for her husband who has dementia)

The most common reasons given by carers for telling the person with dementia their diagnosis are that the person had asked, and to provide an explanation for their experiences. Withholding information occurred when the carer felt disclosure would cause distress, such as anxiety, depression or anger. Another major reason was that the person with dementia was too cognitively impaired to understand. A small number of carers may believe that the diagnosis was wrong (Heal and Husband 1998; Husband 1996). It has been suggested by Meyers (1997) that it is important for people to know the diagnosis so as to be able to 'set their affairs in order' by making a will, an advance decision or drawing up a lasting power of attorney.

There are interesting differences in people's attitudes to disclosure in relation to themselves and others. A study in a memory clinic found that 83 per cent of people attending with a relative did not wish that relative to be told of a dementia diagnosis. However, 71 per cent would wish to know if they themselves were to develop dementia (Maguire *et al.* 1996). In a study of cognitively intact adults in a primary care setting, almost all, 91.9 per cent, indicated they would wish to be told if they were diagnosed with a dementia disorder (Erde, Nadal and Scholl 1988). The Heal and Husband study (1998) found that 58 per cent of carers would wish to know if they were diagnosed with dementia, with a further 15 per cent being unsure. The 58 per cent of carers were significantly more likely to have disclosed the diagnosis to the person they cared for.

Carers need to be consulted where possible about disclosure issues, even though a health professional may have to override their wishes, for example when the person with dementia expresses a desire to talk about the diagnosis. Few carers get the opportunity to discuss the pros and cons of disclosure with a health professional. Where professionals have told the diagnosis, in about 8 per cent of cases the carers felt the outcome of this was negative, in particular when it resulted in angry denial and accusations of betrayal. It is important to remember that it is the carer, not the health professional, who will live with the consequences of disclosure.

How do people cope with knowing they have dementia?

> It is really important for me to know what is going on, I want doctors to tell me what is happening, I want to have a voice, not be treated as though what I have to say does not matter. (Vera, a 66-year-old woman with a diagnosis of Alzheimer's disease)

Being told that one has dementia is a major negative life event. The person with dementia has to cope not only with their fears in relation to the course of the disorder but with the stigma attached to the dementia label. We should expect anxiety and preoccupation, some degree of adaptation reaction being essentially normal.

It should be recognised that diagnostic disclosure is not an event, but a process. By the time the diagnosis is made it should be a matter of confirming to an individual that they have dementia, rather than it being a 'bolt from the blue'. This process should begin as soon as the person presents to services. Probing questions should be asked to ascertain the degree to which the person suspects or fears they have dementia, their understanding of what is happening to them and the importance they attach to it. People may need repeated opportunities to talk about these things and often do not disclose their fears until a trusting relationship has been established. When people deny or minimise their problems it is particularly important to discuss this with relatives, to get their view on the person's level of insight and desire to be given information. Health professionals need to ensure they do not collude with minimisation and to explain what tests such as neuropsychological assessment and MRI scans can and cannot show.

A small study of ten newly diagnosed people found that the most prominent worry in relation to the diagnosis was other people finding out (Husband 2000). They described fears of being pitied, feeling ashamed and humiliated by the diagnosis and others laughing at them. This was related to equally prominent fears of letting oneself down in public. People were worried they might do something embarrassing, appear stupid, incompetent or boring. Fears were also expressed at the prospect of increasing disability and being a burden on others. Of the sample, seven people feared that they would no longer be consulted and decisions would be made for them. They thought that others would think they were incapable of knowing what they wanted. Participants also had individual worries, such as the woman who lived in an isolated rural village and had been told she must stop driving and the man who feared his younger wife would leave him.

The response to the need to maintain secrecy was in all cases a restriction of social activity. People ceased previously enjoyed social activities and avoided all but close friends. This was particularly the case for activities where a skill was being used such as singing in a choir or taking minutes at a meeting. Relatives and close friends were asked to maintain secrecy. People described avoiding situations where their dementia was known about, such as doctors' surgeries and hospitals. A second common effect was for people to become hypervigilant about their own memory function. Memory lapses tended to be maximised and successes minimised. Any lapse increased anxiety and provoked catastrophic thoughts about progression. The negative effects of anxiety on memory function are well known: the more anxious the person, the worse their memory.

On the positive side people who learned their diagnosis reported some relief at knowing there was an explanation for their problems. Some had wondered if they were 'going mad' or imagining the problem. People reported that it helped to focus on short-term goals and over half were using 'alternative remedies' such as ginko biloba (prescription drugs for slowing the course of dementia were unavailable in the area at the time this study was done). Being able to talk to close friends or family about what they would like for the future was also reassuring for most people.

Does telling the diagnosis present an opportunity for intervention?

> I used to get so wound up if I couldn't do something, I would sit and cry as if it was the end of the world. Now I make myself go in the garden, walk away and come back later. What does it matter if I can't bake a cake? Anyway, when I've calmed down I can often do it. (Joan, a 69-year-old woman with dementia)

One issue that must be addressed as we move toward a more open approach to disclosure is the availability of support post diagnosis. Until recently there has been an almost complete absence of counselling available for those newly diagnosed with dementia. Although the needs of people with dementia and their carers for information, advice and emotional support may overlap, it must be acknowledged that separate needs may also exist.

Not everybody with dementia needs individual counselling, but they do need information about their condition, including sensitive discussion of the prognosis. They need to understand how their cognitive problems affect daily life, and consider simple strategies to minimise the impact of these problems. They may need to discuss worries about driving or other independence issues. There are questions relating to what to tell other people and coping with social situations. There may be issues relating to finance or benefit entitlement.

Of equal importance are the emotional issues. How can people be helped to maintain their self-esteem and feelings of self-efficacy after the diagnosis is made? People with dementia have to cope with the loss of independence and competence and face increasing dependency. Support and encouragement are needed to help people focus on the things they can still enjoy, to derive a sense of achievement and to challenge their own self-stigmatising beliefs. For those who become anxious and depressed, individual or group therapy tailored to their specific needs may be considered (see Chapters 7 and 9 of this book).

Despite assumptions that cognitive impairment presents too great an obstacle to engagement with, or understanding of, the therapeutic process, psychological approaches have been used for people with dementia. An exploratory study using cognitive behaviour therapy with people with mild to moderate dementia in the USA found it useful in overcoming depressive withdrawal and catastrophisation (Teri and Gallagher-Thompson 1991; Thompson *et al*. 1990). The issues of loss and grieving have been usefully addressed by psychodynamic psychotherapy (e.g. Hausman 1992; Solomon and Szwabo 1992). Support groups for people with dementia and counselling about diagnosis are becoming more commonly available in western societies (Barton *et al*. 2001; Hawkins and Eagger 1998; Yale 1998). Recent work has demonstrated the potential benefits of cognitive behavioural therapy to enhance mood and psychosocial adjustment and cognitive rehabilitation to aid adaptation and adjustment to cognitive decline (Clare *et al*. 2000; Clare and Woods 2001; Husband 1999; Kipling, Bailey and Charlesworth 1999). A review paper by Cheston (1998) discusses the issues raised for therapists using psychological approaches with people with dementia (see Chapter 9 of this book).

Case example – Jacquie

Jacquie was referred to services at the relatively young age of 57 years complaining of problems with her memory and organisational skills. She worked full time as a practice nurse at a busy rural health centre and was having problems with managing computer records, the administration of clinics and remembering personal information about her patients (such as the names of their children or their jobs). She had recently found immense difficulty preparing the Christmas dinner for her extended family, despite this being a task she had managed very successfully for years. She was anxious she might make a mistake at work and so had taken sick leave.

Jacquie initially believed she might have a brain tumour although the neurological investigations quickly ruled this out. When she received a diagnosis of Alzheimer's disease she described herself as 'only half prepared'. Her first action was to resign from her job by letter, sending her husband to collect her belongings. She was firmly of the opinion that she did want to know her diagnosis, but felt she had been told in an insensitive way which did not encourage information seeking, or offer any hope or reassurance. She had not told either of her sons or any other friends and family about the diagnosis and was avoiding social contact whenever possible. She had been offered a trial of the anti-dementia drug donepezil, but was undecided about this as she felt there was no point. She described an inability to enjoy anything, lack of motivation and a feeling of numbness. She made a new will, an *advance decision* and drew up a lasting power of attorney shortly after hearing the diagnosis.

Jacquie was referred for some psychological intervention to help her manage the impact of the diagnosis. She initially presented with profound feelings of hopelessness with well-elaborated fears for the future. She experienced frequent intrusive thoughts and imagery about being in a residential care home, highly distressed, in an advanced state of dementia. She also described feelings of anger and 'why me?' She felt distressed whenever she thought about the diagnosis or was reminded of it in any way. She had refused antidepressants.

The aim of the intervention was to explore Jacquie's understanding of dementia, her responses to the diagnosis and to help her to develop a coping framework. She was encouraged to explore her thoughts and beliefs about dementia, for example, her ideas about long-term care being imminent and necessarily distressing. She was helped to find out about her condition and in doing so realised that it could be many years before she reached that level of disability. She had some misinformation stemming from past experience as a nurse many years ago. It was suggested to her that we needed to develop a collaborative plan aimed at keeping her functioning as well as possible for as long as possible. It was at this point that she decided taking donepezil could be a useful part of an overall coping strategy. A Mini Mental State Examination carried out before commencement of drug therapy yielded a score of 30/30, which she found reassuring (Folstein, Folstein and McHugh 1975).

Jacquie had to learn to manage her own level of activity and demand. If she set the social and intellectual demands of her daily schedule too high, she became very tired and was failure prone. Too low, and she experienced boredom, frustration and 'feeling stupid'. It was suggested that sharing the diagnosis with other family members and close friends could be a good thing, as trying to cover up cognitive problems was exhausting and led to social withdrawal. She was encouraged to pace her activities and not cram too much into one day, to carry out one task at a time and to spend time planning her activities. She was asked to continue activities she knew she could manage, particularly if they were sources of enjoyment. She also recorded activities she was finding difficult and we identified what help she would need were she to continue to do them. Her husband joined in some of these sessions as he was usually the 'help provider'. Finally, it was suggested she join the local younger people with dementia group run by the Alzheimer's Society.

Jacquie gradually felt less catastrophic about her diagnosis and that she had more control over her well-being. She still feared for the future, but these fears were more realistic and less overwhelming. She responded well to the donepezil and intended to continue with it for as long as it proved useful. The elements of the intervention described here are mainly based on a simplified version of cognitive behaviour therapy (Beck et al. 1979).

Conclusion

Being open with people about diagnosis presents a real opportunity for health professionals to intervene early, both to prevent problems and to help with problems as they arise. Improving our dialogue with people with dementia allows us to think and respond more appropriately to the challenges of dementia care. It is to be hoped that establishing openness and trust early on will facilitate good future relationships with services. We now need more research to look at the impact of counselling or psychological therapy over the longer term, and to examine the processes within interventions that are helpful.

References

Barton, J., Piney, C., Berg, M. and Parker, C. (2001) 'Coping with Forgetfulness Group.' *PSIGE – Psychology Specialists Promoting Psychological Wellbeing in Late Life – Newsletter 77*, 19–25.

Beck, A.T., Rush, A.J., Shaw, B.F. and Emery, G. (1979) *The Cognitive Therapy of Depression*. New York, NY: Guilford Press.

Cheston, R. (1998) 'Psychotherapeutic work with people with dementia: a review of the literature.' *British Journal of Medical Psychology 71*, 211–231.

Clare, L., Wilson, B.A., Carter, G., Breen, E.K., Gosses, A. and Hodges, J.R. (2000) 'Intervening with everyday memory problems in dementia of the Alzheimer's type: an errorless learning approach.' *Journal of Clinical and Experimental Neuropsychology 22*, 132–146.

Clare, L. and Woods, R.T. (2001) *Cognitive Rehabilitation in Dementia*. Hove: Psychology Press.

Erde, E., Nadal, E. and Scholl, T. (1988) 'On truth telling and the diagnosis of Alzheimer's disease.' *Journal of Family Practice 26*, 401–406.

Folstein, M.F., Folstein, S.E. and McHugh, P.R. (1975) 'Mini-mental state: a practical method for grading the cognitive state of patients for the clinician.' *Journal of Psychiatric Research 12*, 607–614.

Gilliard, J. and Gwilliam, C. (1996) 'Sharing the diagnosis: a survey of memory disorders clinics, their policies on informing people and their families and the support they offer.' *International Journal of Geriatric Psychiatry 11*, 1001–1003.

Gillon, R. (1985) 'Telling the truth and medical ethics.' *British Medical Journal 291*, 1556–1557.

Hausman, C.D. (1992) 'Dynamic Psychotherapy with Elderly Demented Patients.' In G. Jones and B. Mieson (eds) *Caregiving in Dementia*. London: Routledge.

Hawkins, D. and Eagger, S. (1998) 'Group therapy: sharing the pain of diagnosis.' *Journal of Dementia Care 6*, 12–14.

Heal, H.C. and Husband, H.J. (1998) 'Disclosing a diagnosis of dementia: is age a factor?' *Aging and Mental Health 2*, 144–150.

Husband, H.J. (1996) 'Sharing the diagnosis – how do carers feel?' *Journal of Dementia Care 4*, 18–20.

Husband, H.J. (1999) 'The psychological consequences of learning of a dementia diagnosis: three case examples.' *Aging and Mental Health 3*, 179–183.

Husband, H.J. (2000) 'Diagnostic disclosure in dementia: an opportunity for intervention?' *International Journal of Geriatric Psychiatry 15*, 544–547.

Kipling, T., Bailey, M. and Charlesworth, G. (1999) 'The feasibility of a cognitive behavioural therapy group for men with mild/moderate impairment.' *Behavioural and Cognitive Psychotherapy 27*, 189–193.

Kitwood, T. (1997) 'The experience of dementia.' *Aging and Mental Health 1*, 13–23.

Maguire, C.P., Kirby, M., Coen, R., Coakley, D., Lawler, B.A. and O'Neil, D. (1996) 'Family members' attitudes toward telling the patient with Alzheimer's disease their diagnosis.' *British Medical Journal 314*, 375–376.

Meyers, B.S. (1997) 'Telling patients they have Alzheimer's disease.' *British Medical Journal 314*, 321–322.

Novak, D.H., Plumer, R., Smith, R.L., Ochitill, H., Morrow, G.R. and Bennett, J.M. (1979) 'Changes in physicians' attitudes toward telling the cancer patient.' *Journal of the American Medical Association 241*, 897–900.

Oken, D. (1961) 'What to tell cancer patients.' *Journal of the American Medical Association 175*, 1120–1128.

Rice, K. and Warner, N. (1994) 'Breaking the bad news: what do psychiatrists tell patients with dementia about their illness?' *International Journal of Geriatric Psychiatry 9*, 467–471.

Solomon, K. and Szwabo, P. (1992) 'Psychotherapy for People with Dementia.' In J.E. Morley, R.M. Coe, R. Strong and G.T. Grossberg (eds) *Memory Functions and Ageing Related Disorders.* New York, NY: Springer.

Teri, L. and Gallagher-Thompson, D. (1991) 'Cognitive behavioral intervention for the treatment of depression in Alzheimer's patients.' *Gerontologist 31*, 413–416.

Thompson, L.W., Wenger, G., Zeuss, J.D. and Gallagher, D. (1990) 'CBT with early stage Alzheimer's Disease Patients: An Exploratory View of the Utility of this Approach.' In E. Light and B.D. Lebowitz (eds) *Alzheimer's Disease – Treatment and Family Stress.* New York, NY: Hemisphere.

Vassilas, C.A. (1999) 'How often do GPs tell people with dementia about the truth about their diagnosis?' *Alzheimer's Disease Society National Newsletter*, February 1999, 5.

Yale, R. (1998) *Developing Support Groups for Individuals with Early-stage Alzheimer's Disease.* Baltimore, MD: Health Professions Press.

Further reading and related references

Bamford, C., Lamont, S., Eccles, M., Robinson, L., May, C. and Bond, J. (2004) 'Disclosing a diagnosis of dementia: a systematic review.' *International Journal of Geriatric Psychiatry 19*, 151–169.

De Lepeleire, J. and Heyrman, J. (1999) 'Diagnosis and management of dementia in primary care at an early stage: the need for a new concept and an adapted procedure.' *Theoretical Medicine and Bioethics 20*, 215–228.

Pratt, R. and Wilkinson, H. (2003) 'A psychosocial model of understanding the experience of receiving a diagnosis of dementia.' *Dementia 2*, 181–199.

Robinson, L., Clare, L. and Evans, K. (2005) 'Making sense of dementia and adjusting to loss: psychological reactions to a diagnosis of dementia in couples.' *Aging and Mental Health 9*, 337–347.

Wilkinson, H. and Milne, A.J. (2003) 'Sharing a diagnosis of dementia – learning from the patient perspective.' *Aging and Mental Health 7*, 300–307.

Chapter 3

Timely Psychosocial Interventions in a Memory Clinic

Esme Moniz-Cook, Gillian Gibson,
Jas Harrison and Hannah Wilkinson

Overview

This chapter describes interventions to prevent or minimise disability and distress in early dementia. The programme described was developed during two controlled psychosocial intervention memory clinic studies and provides protocols that promote health and psychosocial well-being in older people with suspected dementia. First, the results and implications of the two studies are summarised. Then a rationale for the programme protocols is presented. Finally, four protocols are outlined:

- to provide a communication strategy for separating neurological impairment from quality of life, following a memory assessment

- to promote health

- to pre-empt the negative impact of cognitive losses on functional independence, by maintaining purpose, pleasure and valued relationships

- to support family members.

We make use of anonymised case study illustrations to demonstrate how the protocols may relate to individuals.

Background: early psychosocial intervention 'memory clinic' studies

This programme was developed within controlled and implementation studies that span over a decade in a UK memory clinic. Following memory clinic assessment, the first study provided an in-home individualised psychosocial intervention, using cognitive rehabilitation methods that included families in supporting their relative in the use of external memory aids over a three-month period. At six-month follow-up, these carers were more distressed compared with the treatment-as-usual group (Moniz-Cook et al. 1998). However by 18-month follow-up, the treatment had a positive effect on memory in people with early dementia (F = 14.49, df = 1,28, p = 0.001), as well as on carer depression (F = 17.03, df = 1,18, p = 0.001) and carer anxiety (F = 15.58, df = 1,18, p = 0.001). In addition, more people with dementia in treatment group were still living in their own homes.

In a second study, in addition to behavioural activation (pleasurable activity), health promotion and carer support, interventions were added to the original cognitive rehabilitation programme to provide home-based multi-component psychosocial intervention for people with suspected dementia and their families. Slightly increased levels of distress in carers at six months, compared with treatment-as-usual, were noted (Moniz-Cook et al. 2001a, 2001b). However, this time the effect was not marked, probably due to inclusion of the additional programme protocols, which may have moderated carer distress over the initial intervention period. This second study also demonstrated positive outcomes over time, where at 12-month follow-up people with dementia were less depressed (F = 7.870, df =1,42, p = 0.0076), carers reported fewer memory and behaviour problems (F = 8.883, df = 1,42, p = 0.0048), improved coping ability (F = 6.84, df = 1,41, p = 0.0124) and more people with dementia were cared for at home.

The impact of early psychosocial intervention in early dementia on family members is not well understood. For example, in one UK study families have reported high satisfaction with a 7-week memory remediation group offered to their relative with early dementia (James and Sabin 2005), but the consequence was that they began to focus on their relatives' deficits and thus progressed to assuming a 'care-giving role'. An early memory remediation group for people with suspected dementia and family carers also reported negative effects on carer mood (Zarit, Zarit and Reever 1982), as did a group-based educational support programme for family carers (Russell, Proctor and Moniz-Cook 1989), which appeared to exacerbate anxieties about the future or prognosis and dementia-related deterioration. Being aware of the risk of reduced mood or depression among family carers during early psychosocial intervention programmes is important, as carer mood is a good predictor of family participation and adherence to in-home interventions (Gitlin *et al.* 1999).

In the two studies described above, the potential for developing mood problems over time may have been reduced by regular contact by the practitioner with the person and their family, after the initial three-month implementation of in-home psychosocial intervention. Further support for this conclusion is seen in a study where families whose relatives with early dementia received group-based day hospital intervention over a 12-month period reported high satisfaction with this, but their mood significantly worsened, compared with equivalent groups where carers and their relatives received in-home or outpatient psychosocial treatments (Richards *et al.* 2003). What these studies show is that families are an important part of the person with dementia's social context and that the impact of a psychosocial intervention will be influenced by this context. Therefore, the person and the carer, as well as other supporting family and friends, will need to engage with the aims of psychosocial intervention. To properly focus an intervention requires assessment of personal circumstances, relationships, concerns and hopes of both person with dementia and their family (see Moniz-Cook 2008, for a framework for assessment).

Rationale

The early intervention programmes used in the studies above have their conceptual and empirical basis within:

- models of psychosocial disability in dementia (Gilliard *et al.* 2005)
- paradigms of health promotion (Naidoo and Willis 2000; Nutbeam 1998)
- psychosocial well-being.

We suggest that the aims of psychosocial interventions in a memory clinic are helpfully set within the paradigm of health promotion. These may be described as 'secondary health promoting interventions' (see Naidoo and Willis 2000) since they are early interventions that attempt to postpone progression of a condition (in this case we have translated this to mean *progressive disabilities*) and thus maintain well-being. In working with people with early dementia, the aims may be:

- to prevent future distress by addressing the longer term sources of 'excess disabilities' (Sabat 1994), i.e. the extra health and psychosocial disabilities commonly seen in older people with suspected dementia that are not directly related to brain damage or cognitive loss

- to promote maintenance of purpose, pleasure, meaningful activity, valued relationships and quality of life.

Therefore the prophylactic function of intervention, i.e. strategies for preventing distress and disability and promoting health and psychosocial well-being, is implicit within our defined aims of early intervention in dementia. Furthermore interventions may be offered irrespective of a dementia diagnosis, including when this is uncertain, where a 'watching brief' is needed or where mild cognitive impairment is present.

'Prevention' and health promotion in early dementia

In recent years the notion of 'preventable dementia' has arisen in the context of Vascular Cognitive Impairment (VCI) (Bowler and Hachinski 2003), Mild Cognitive Impairment (MCI) (Tuokko and Hultsch 2006) and epidemiological evidence of risk factors, neuro-protection and enhancing of neuronal reserves (Purandare, Ballard and Burns 2005). From this literature the treatment of vascular risk factors such as hypertension, high cholesterol, diabetes, narrowing of the main arteries to the brain, heart disease and smoking are all identified as important preventative strategies and these can continue to apply to older people with early dementia. Similarly, strategies for neuro-protection in the prevention of dementia – such as treatment for levels of folate and vitamin B_{12} or antioxidants (Vitamins C and E and alcohol), are equally applicable when a dementia diagnosis has been reached. For example, reduced serum vitamin B_{12} may predispose people with frontotemporal dementia to develop hallucinations and sleep disturbances (Engelborghs *et al.* 2004). The third area of interest in preventing dementia is what has been described as 'enhancing of neuronal reserves' – often in middle age – by increasing cognitive, physical and pleasurable social activity (Purandare *et al.* 2005). There is an emerging empirical basis for this notion in early dementia. For example, there is some evidence that people with Alzheimer's disease can compensate for cognitive loss in one area of the brain by increased activity in another brain region (Grady 2007); cognitive stimulation can postpone cognitive decline in dementia (Spector *et al.* 2003); and proactive physical and pleasurable social activity can moderate mood decline in people with dementia (Eggermont and Scherder 2006; Moniz-Cook *et al.* 2001a, 2001b; Teri *et al.* 1997) and their carers (Moniz-Cook *et al.* 1998, 2001a, 2001b; Teri *et al.* 1997).

The health promotion literature outlines risks to functional independence, health and well-being in older people, including medication effects and injurious falls (Nutbeam 1998). Common medications associated with falls include narcotic painkillers, anticonvulsants and antidepressants (Kelly *et al.* 2003) or sedatives and hypnotics (Oliver *et al.* 2004). The health promotion strategy for early dementia developed in the present early intervention programme in the memory clinic described here did the following:

- monitored the known risk factors for developing dementia and provided timely treatment when needed

- addressed the known risks (particularly falls, medication prescription and medicine management) for functional dependency in older people

- monitored and provided psychosocial intervention when needed, such as cognitive, physical and pleasurable social activity to maintain psychosocial well-being.

The person's family physician (general practitioner, GP) acted as joint case manager with the memory clinic practitioner (Moniz-Cook, Gibson and Win 1997), in the delivery of the programme.

'Prevention' and psychosocial disability in memory clinics

The introductory chapter of this book outlines the powerful impact of the double stigma of age and dementia, which for many older people brings with it fears of loss of control and misunderstandings of what could be achieved to moderate or postpone distress and disability. This can have a subtle but important effect on the potential for older people attending a memory clinic and their families to engage with health-promoting and psychosocial interventions that protect against the known negative consequences of a suspected dementia on well-being and quality of life.

Some practices in specialist outpatient memory clinics can, we suggest, undermine engagement of older people and families in programmes to promote health and psychosocial well-being. For example, protocols of pre-diagnostic counselling, requiring a person to decide whether they wish to be told their diagnosis or not – at a time when she or he may have only just tentatively decided that it is worth exploring what is on offer to overcome, as yet, unexpressed fears (Moniz-Cook *et al.* 2006) – may serve to reinforce the documented fears of loss of control in first-time memory clinic attendees. Post-diagnostic protocols for acetylcholinesterase inhibitor (AChEI) medications, information on matters such as lasting power of attorney (in England and Wales), *advance decisions,* social security benefits, driving, issues of safety and signposting to local and national organisations have their place, but they too can sometimes undermine active engagement in proactive collaborative psychosocial interventions. Where memory clinics have been established primarily for evaluation of AChEI medications and these are not suitable for the individual, other forms of protective interventions may be hard to achieve due to disappointed family carers (Moniz-Cook *et al.* 1997) or under-resourced or skill-deficient practitioners and protocols. Finally, if family anxieties are not addressed at the start, family members may inadvertently undermine or not actively support activities that promote health and well-being.

The Hull Memory Clinic early intervention protocols

The psychosocial disability dementia care model (Gilliard *et al.* 2005) suggests that early psychosocial approaches should: focus on remaining abilities and attend to the use of language to avoid negative stereotyping; provide activities that promote autonomy; normalise or personalise activity support by basing this on knowledge of past pleasures, values and interests; and provide a gatekeeping function to prevent others – such as families and professionals – from undermining access to interventions by the person with dementia. Four protocols were developed for psychosocial care in the Hull Memory Clinic. These were explicitly designed sequentially: to neutralise stigma at the time of assessment; to promote health and psychosocial well-being; to support family members. They reflect a multicomponent longitudinal dementia disease 'self-management' programme and, as is common for many secondary health promoting interventions (Naidoo and Willis 2000), are set at the interface of primary and secondary community-based care.

The programme comprises four parts, delivered consecutively:

1. A meeting with the person and family to discuss the memory tests.

2. An invitation to them and their wider family and friends to attend a half-day workshop on 'Understanding and Coping with Memory as You Get Older' (see Box 3.1).

3. Between six and eight in-home or outpatient treatment sessions over 12 months to provide components of the psychosocial intervention.

4. After 12 months, a system of longitudinal tracking, with support where needed, from the memory clinic practitioner and the GP. Longitudinal tracking refers to a primary care strategy that allows a 'condition specific' case manager to routinely monitor people with long-term health conditions.

In the studies described earlier each person with early dementia was 'case managed' in primary care by a memory clinic practitioner and the person's GP (Moniz-Cook *et al.* 1997), unless the person or the family carer became significantly distressed or respite and/or long-term care was required. In these instances, the person was referred on to specialist mental health and social care services. In the UK these are usually co-ordinated and delivered within secondary (i.e. community-based teams) or tertiary (i.e. psychiatric in-patient hospital) care.

A language for separating neurological impairment from quality of life

The memory assessment can be used to focus on remaining abilities and avoid negative stereotyping by:

- clarifying the person's strengths and how these may be maximised

- explaining the sources of reported memory concerns

- providing compensatory strategies for particular difficulties due to cognitive loss.

Three methods were used in the Hull Memory Clinic, following memory testing. Each were aimed at reinforcing cognitive strengths, outlining how these may be maximised, providing explanations for reported memory concerns and advising on compensatory strategies. The psychologist first used a simplified illustration of cognitive function (the 'cognitive map', see Figure 3.1) for all patients and their families at the post-memory assessment meeting. Then, where requested, a written summary of advice for concerns raised at the family meeting (see Figure 3.2) was provided. Finally, families were invited to a monthly half-day workshop to reinforce the principles of cognitive rehabilitation (Box 3.1) which formed the basis of the first psychosocial intervention component described later. The case studies of Donald, Fleur and Sandra that follow illustrate how each of these methods worked in practice.

Box 3.1 Family Workshop: 'Understanding and Coping with Memory as You Get Older'

WHAT IS MEMORY?

- Immediate/working; Long term; and Prospective Memory.

Exercises on each of these, for example: *What was the number we showed you a few minutes ago?* (immediate memory).

- Semantic (memory for facts); Episodic/autobiographical (personal information); and Procedural/implicit (skills) Memory.

Exercises on each of these, for example: *What is the capital of France?* (facts); *What did you have for breakfast?* (episodic memory); *Tie your shoe laces* (procedural/implicit memory).

- Verbal and Visual Memory.

Exercises on each of these, for example: *What is the name of the consultant?* (verbal memory); *What colour is the receptionist's hair?* (visual memory).

- Recall and Recognition Memory.

Exercises on each of these, for example: *Who was the famous cinema actress who married Prince Rainier of Monaco?* (recall); *Who in the room have you seen before today? Who is the lady in this photograph?* (recognition memory).

- Stages of the Memory Process
  - Encoding (taking in or registering information)
  - Storage (retaining)
  - Retrieval (getting it out again).

OTHER COGNITIVE FUNCTIONS

- Language – speech and comprehension
- Perception
- Praxis – voluntary control of movement
- Executive functions.

COMPENSATING FOR MEMORY – RELATED PROBLEMS

- Pros and cons to the idea of *'Use it or Lose it'*
- Why external memory aids?
- A review of strategies to compensate for particular memory problems
- Efficient strategies for learning new things.

Case example – Donald

Donald, aged 78, was diagnosed with Alzheimer's disease some four years ago and had maintained a relatively active life until recently. His wife reported that he had now become clumsy, often knocking teacups over, and that he was unsteady on his feet resulting in a series of recent falls. This had impacted on his life as he had lost the confidence to go out for walks or tend to his garden. She believed that he was now too frail to engage in such activities and he had become fearful of falling. The consequence was that he had become depressed. An assessment suggested particular new difficulties with depth perception, probably due to infarction (since people with Alzheimer's disease can also develop vascular-related memory complaints) rather than frailty per se. The simplified cognitive map (Figure 3.1) was used to explain to Donald and his family the potential cause of the reported concerns. Once reassured, he and his family engaged in rehabilitation to compensate for this. Later he used similar strategies to overcome his 'clumsiness'. Donald's understandable fears of falling were addressed with fall-preventive strategies. He thus returned to going out for his regular walks and gardening and reported that he was now much happier in himself.

Case example – Fleur

Fleur, aged 78, was an active person who attended the memory clinic because her husband John was convinced that she had Alzheimer's disease and wished to access drugs (i.e. the AChEIs) that might help her with this. Fleur herself was not keen on any drugs – 'let alone drugs for the mind'. She felt that her memory 'was fine'. Fleur and John had used the internet to find out about dementia diagnoses before attending the clinic. They both agreed that in the past three months she had become somewhat hesitant and lacking in confidence, particularly with activities in the home. John felt that he now had to do more to assist with preparation of meals and some household tasks. Fleur had also recently decided to stop driving and discontinue her insurance for their joint car. During the post-assessment meeting with them, a diagnosis of vascular dementia was discussed. John remained keen that his wife was offered an AChEI and since she was not eligible for this in the UK National Health Service, he wished to pay for it. Fleur did not want to take drugs and, having outlined her day-to-day concerns, she requested a written summary of the meeting (Figure 3.2) for her to discuss with their son and daughter-in law, who were not present. Their son attended the half-day workshop (see Box 3.1) with his mother and encouraged his father in providing day-to-day support for Fleur, as they used in-home cognitive rehabilitation to compensate for her day-to-day memory difficulties. John continued to feel that his wife would benefit from a drug, but nonetheless supported her in her efforts to maintain her pleasurable social activities, including dropping her off to activities that did not involve him, such as choir practice.

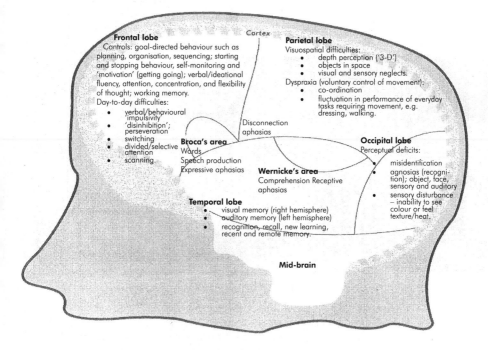

Figure 3.1 Using a simplified 'cognitive map' to discuss the memory assessment

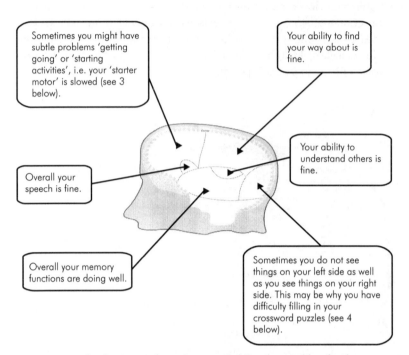

Sometimes you might have subtle problems 'getting going' or 'starting activities', i.e. your 'starter motor' is slowed (see 3 below).

Your ability to find your way about is fine.

Your ability to understand others is fine.

Overall your speech is fine.

Overall your memory functions are doing well.

Sometimes you do not see things on your left side as well as you see things on your right side. This may be why you have difficulty filling in your crossword puzzles (see 4 below).

Figure 3.2 Example of written information provided for Fleur and her family

Here are some explanations to the questions you raised with us at our meeting.

1. **What are TIAs/mini strokes?** Transient ischemic attacks (TIAs) and 'mini strokes' are the second most common cause of memory difficulties in people over 65. They occur when a part of the brain is temporarily deprived of its blood supply, which carries oxygen to the brain. They may occur suddenly and last for quite short periods – between 5 and 30 minutes and much less in the case of a TIA. Sometimes people may not be aware they are happening (particularly as in the case of a TIA); others may be aware of 'strange sensations'; and in other cases temporary problems such as double vision, numbness, weakness or tingling in an arm, leg, hand or foot and dizziness are reported. Mostly people feel they have 'recovered' from these episodes after a period of time. Mini stroke can affect any part of the brain – in your case they have generally affected functioning towards the back of the brain. This means that most of the brain is working fairly normally for your age and some parts of the brain may also sometimes take over the function of parts where complete recovery from the mini stroke has not occurred. Some of the concerns you have raised with us are where you are noticing the impact of mini stroke (see below – 3 and 4).

2. **How can I stop things from getting worse?** We have advised your GP to consider prescribing aspirin to thin your blood and thus reduce the likelihood of a further mini stroke. It is important however, that you *do not* start taking any medication without your GP's consent, as certain medication (including aspirin)

could interfere with your general health. Having high blood pressure can make things worse but your GP has already prescribed you with medication to lower your blood pressure. You should ensure that you attend surgery regularly for blood pressure checks and at least once a year for blood tests to check that you have not developed new conditions such as anaemia, diabetes and so on. Alcohol needs to be kept to a minimum as excessive alcohol, like fat and salt, raises blood pressure. Since you are hypertensive it may also be a good idea to slightly reduce your caffeine (coffee and tea) intake. You are therefore advised to eat a well-balanced diet, which is low in fat and salt. Exercise can also help so check with your GP about sources of advice for this or book into one of our Active Lifestyles Consultations at our drop-in-centre. Going for a regular 15–20 minute walk each day is probably all you need for now, but take care on pavements (see 4 below).

3. **Why do I have trouble 'getting going'?** You may find that sometimes you have difficulty putting your thoughts into action. Although you may know exactly how to do something and can describe it to others, you have difficulty carrying out the action or activity. You may find that you have difficulty starting an activity, i.e. your 'starter motor' is slow. Sometimes this can make other people think that you are 'hesitant' or have lost confidence or are being slow, but it is important to recognise that this is not the case. If this occurs, try asking your husband to physically prompt you to get going on a task – as we have demonstrated to you at clinic, once you have got going, you won't have too much trouble continuing with what you want do.

4. **Why do I have difficulty filling in my crosswords?** Our tests showed that often you see things better on your right side than your left side. You are already compensating for this by moving things around until you can see them properly and you should continue to do this as it is a very good strategy. For the same reason you may: (a) bump into things more easily such as doors or furniture because although your eyesight is fine, you might occasionally 'miss' or 'misperceive' parts of your environment; (b) become at risk of stumbling or tripping over kerbs, paving stones or rugs. These and times when you are getting in and out of chairs/beds or using the toilet/bath can unfortunately precipitate a fall. We will discuss with you and your husband ways in which you may reduce the risk of falls when we visit you at home.

5. **Should I stop any of my social activities?** It is vital that you *do not* stop or withdraw from the social activities/hobbies that you currently engage in even though you may now be embarrassed at the apparent 'mistakes' you make. With respect to the social activities that you enjoy with your family and friends it is a case of adopting the policy of 'use it or lose it' as they provide you with important mental stimulation. Do things with people you trust – they will overlook your occasional mistake and encourage you to keep going. Do continue with your choir, weekly dancing, contact with your grandchildren, attending classical concerts and theatre and other activities.

Case example – Sandra

Sandra, aged 67, had lived with her daughter Brenda for the last 20 years and had supported her in raising her sons and managing the home. She reported that she was concerned about her declining memory. Brenda did not feel that her mother had memory problems but that she had become increasingly 'lazy' and had, for example, lost interest in the house. Brenda felt that she had to constantly 'nag' at her mother to do things. They both agreed that this had led to increasing tension in the household. The memory assessment indicated that Sandra was developing what psychologists refer to as 'dysexecutive syndrome', where more than one of the cognitive deficits associated with the front of the brain (Figure 3.1) were noted, including difficulties with task initiation. In contrast, most aspects of memory function were relatively unimpaired. The simplified 'cognitive map' was used to explain to Sandra and Brenda the consequences of deficits associated with 'dysexecutive syndrome', including how reduced 'initiation' can affect a person's ability to do things that they wish to. Brenda remained sceptical and decided to await outcome of the MRI scan which was underway. In the meantime she and her mother attended the half-day workshop where Sandra (see previous case) and her son were also present. They had grasped the concept of difficulty in initiating tasks due to 'starter motor problems' and described their successes in overcoming the effects of this using the advice provided (see Figure 3.2). This motivated Brenda to take advantage of rehabilitation techniques to prompt initiation and thus assist her mother in increasing her activity around the home. Subsequently Sandra was diagnosed with a frontal-type dementia.

Promoting health in early dementia

The interventions included in this protocol are based on the rationale for health promotion in early dementia outlined previously. The following reviews were routinely applied, usually by a memory nurse, or where available (as noted in brackets below) a relevant primary care professional:

- medication review (pharmacist)

- diet and nutrition review (dietician)

- exercise and physical activity review (therapist)

- risk of injury due to falling review (therapist).

Treatment was provided by the GP who also monitored health status for new conditions such as infection, anaemia and diabetes. The longitudinal tracking system allowed the memory clinic case manager, usually the memory nurse, if needed, to prompt the person and the carer to request review (with a recommended minimum of once a year) by the GP.

Promoting control and pleasure in early dementia

The interventions included in this protocol may be seen as those which enhance neuronal reserves through cognitive, social and leisure activity; i.e. the third group of strategies outlined by Purandare *et al.* (2005, p.176). However, the psychosocial literature on the development of disability in older people with suspected dementia offers a stronger rationale for this protocol, where interventions included can have two separate aims as follows:

1. To provide cognition-orientated activity that promotes a sense of control and autonomy by counteracting the anxieties and fears (Moniz-Cook *et al.* 2006) associated with declining memory in ageing, since anxiety is strongly associated with the progression of disability (Brenes *et al.* 2005).

2. To promote normalisation and social integration (Carter and Everitt 1998), i.e. purposeful, meaningful activity and friendships, since these are core components of positive mental health and well-being and known moderators of hopelessness and depression in old age (Pinquart 2002; Takahasi, Tamura and Tokoro 1997).

Cognition-orientated activity

Three cognitive activity interventions were pursued: two were cognitive rehabilitation interventions and the third provided advice on maximising cognitive strengths such as during conversation, activities of daily living and leisure. These will be outlined next.

1. *Prophylactic cognitive rehabilitation.* This involves training in the use of important external memory aids (see Moniz-Cook *et al.* 1998, Table 1, p.202; Orani *et al.* 2003) aimed at establishing implicit orientation procedures to counteract future decline in prospective and episodic memory. Rehabilitation usually includes the family carer(s) and the psychologist in an active training errorless learning programme based on spaced retrieval techniques (Camp, Bird and Cherry 2000) where goal attainment (i.e. implicit use of external memory aids to support memory) should be reached in a maximum of two weeks. The rationale for this intervention is evidenced in an early study where, as compared with the treatment-as-usual group, the majority of people with early dementia remained at home at 18-month follow-up, since their implicit use of an 'orientation board' allowed

them the control to remain at home without constant supervision
from their family carer (Moniz-Cook *et al.* 1998, p.207). The case of
Bob demonstrates how the wider primary care network may also
support prophylactic use of external memory aids.

Case example – Bob

Bob, aged 77, was a retired company director and an accountant by
profession. His sense of pride lay in his excellent memory which despite
his early dementia did not cause him or his wife problems at present. He
resisted engagement in prophylactic cognitive rehabilitation to establish
implicit orientation procedures, since he believed that this would be the
'lazy way out' and that he needed to 'stimulate his memory by testing it
each day'. In his opinion a cognitive rehabilitation programme was only
necessary if and when his memory worsened. Six months later his GP
conducted a home visit since Bob was feeling 'under the weather'.
During this consultation Bob discovered that his GP, whose opinion he
valued, used memory aids to improve his own memory efficacy.
Encouraged by his GP and with support from his wife and the
psychologist, Bob engaged in prophylactic memory training using
external memory aids of his choice. Bob lived at home with his wife for
eight further years, until he required two months of nursing home
palliative care during the final stages of cancer.

2. *Cognitive rehabilitation* to compensate for, or resolve, current everyday
   concerns for the person (Chapter 4), or more often problems due to
   forgetting reported by adult children whose parent lived alone, such
   as repeated questioning and demanding phone calls (Moniz-Cook *et
   al.* 1998). The case studies of Charles and Mary demonstrate how
   older people living alone can be helped with focused cognitive rehabilitation, to overcome their memory-related problems and remain
   living at home. The strategies and measurement of outcome for these
   cases are found in Moniz-Cook *et al.* (1998, Table 1, p.202).

Case example – Charles

Charles, aged 81, had recently allowed teenage boys known to
experiment with drugs into his home. His son and neighbours were
concerned as Charles insisted on retaining sums of money in the home.
He was a friendly man who was generous to young people such as his
teenage and young adult grandchildren. Charles was an active man
whose functional independence was relatively good. Apart from support
with meal preparation and laundry from his housing provider, he
maintained self-care and enjoyed riding his bike to his allotment. He
attended the memory clinic with his son but insisted that he was fine and

refused to complete the memory tests. In his view entry to residential care for his safety was not an option as 'he would rather be dead, like his brother who had dementia', and had apparently survived only two months following admission to a care home, some years previously. A face recognition programme was established with the cooperation of his neighbour and his son using six familiar and six 'stooge strangers' who initially visited him at home each day. The frequency of visits was graded over eight weeks until he consistently refused entry to strangers over three consecutive weeks. Charles lived at home until his death of a heart attack, some four years later.

Case example – Janet

Janet aged 75, rang her daughter up to 26 times a day, including night-time. Her stressed daughter was convinced that she had dementia, although she was fully functional in the home and despite equivocal findings at the memory clinic where, at the most, Mild Cognitive Impairment of vascular origin (MCI-VaD) was possible. The psychologist established an intensive in-home cognitive rehabilitation programme with the support of her son, who worked abroad but was on home leave with his own family for three weeks. Over a six-week period of intensive training in the use of external memory aids (i.e. a clock with an automatic day and date, used in conjunction with a calendar and a noticeboard for control of prospective memory and a 'memory orientation space' for important items such as her savings book and important letters), Janet's anxious phone calls reduced to three times a day, with no night-time calls, with further improvements to once a day by 12-week follow-up. This was maintained at eight-month follow-up, but four months later Janet was admitted to hospital following a fall whilst out shopping. During this admission her daughter was told that she had dementia and, with support from social services, transfer to a care home was arranged. Janet was agitated at the care home and constantly attempted to leave. She was prescribed sedatives and following a subsequent fall and re-admission to hospital, she suffered a fatal stroke, six weeks later.

3. *Maximising cognitive strengths* using the principles of compensation. Strategies include applying focused attention techniques, reducing cognitive load and maintaining pleasurable mental activity. Examples of these are: using short sentences or closed questions and avoiding pronouns during conversation; reducing the demand for sustained conversation during activities of daily living such as mealtimes; enhancing memory retrieval with visual and verbal cues; and developing personal plans for pleasurable mental activity that are based on past interest and values and are also achievable.

Many of these methods can now be found in texts that have emerged recently (see Clare 2008; Clare and Woods 2001; Hill, Backman and Neely 2002; Woods and Clare 2008).

Purposeful, pleasurable and social activity

Behavioural activation interventions for both the person with dementia and their spouses or partners were used to prevent depression in both, since depressed people with dementia often have depressed family carers (Teri and Truax 1994). Activities should have value, meaning, purpose and provide pleasure for the person and carer. The finding that older people benefit more from social support than behavioural intervention, which if used on their own may be detrimental (Jané-Llopis *et al.* 2002), is an important additional guiding principle for behavioural activation programmes. The Seattle Depression Protocol outlines how this may be achieved (Teri *et al.* 1997; Teri, Lodgson and McCurry 2002, p.647). Methods extracted from the Seattle programme for the Hull-based protocol included:

- scheduling enjoyable activities based on past interests and pleasure, but modifying them if needed

- providing resources such as transport or a volunteer to support the activity

- involving the spouse or partner in the activity where shared pleasure is possible

- using reminiscence including developing life story books and collages (Chapter 11)

- scheduling pleasurable social activity or valued social contact and providing structure for this where opportunities do not exist (Chapter 12).

People with dementia and their spouses found pleasure in a wide range of activities. Examples included 'home making – maintaining the household', going for walks or to the gym, going on holiday, regular singing and dancing sessions with friends, listening to music, joining in pub quizzes, using a computer, having meals with friends, volunteering to assist in a charity shop or a playgroup for children, looking after grandchildren, baking for neighbours, talking to newly diagnosed people with dementia and fund-raising for the Alzheimer's Society. These activities were monitored by the memory clinic case manager within the longitudinal tracking system.

Family carer support

This final protocol provided for the ongoing needs of family caregivers and included the following methods:

- problem solving (Moniz-Cook *et al.* 2008)

- group psycho-educational workshops where carers could attend alone or with their relatives. The workshops comprised advanced strategies as a follow-up to the initial family workshop; communication skills training targeting conversation; and introduction to the principles of emotion-orientated communication where anxieties may be validated to reduce episodes of disorientation (Finnema *et al.* 2000). The final case of Peter and his wife Agnes is an example from one such workshop.

Case example – Peter and Agnes

Peter's wife Agnes was concerned about his visual hallucinations. Peter often mistook his dressing gown, hung on his bedroom door, as a person standing in the bedroom. He was not anxious about this and often 'conversed' with the person. However, Agnes was highly distressed about his 'loss of mind' and worried that he might in the future not know her. The simplified cognitive map was used to explain how occipital lobe damage could contribute to visual disturbances which were often temporarily worse when the brain was overstimulated, such as at night. During the workshop, Irene, daughter of a man with vascular dementia, described how she and her father had, with support from the psychologist, reduced the frequency of such 'misperceptions'. Jeanne, another adult-child carer reported that she had found the book *The Man Who Mistook His Wife for a Hat* (Sachs 1970) helpful in understanding similar difficulties in her mother. Agnes was reassured that her husband's 'hallucinations' were associated with 'tricks of the brain' rather than significant loss of mind.

Conclusions

The psychosocial interventions described in this chapter are focused on the first three steps of the framework for psychosocial intervention in early dementia, suggested in Chapter 1. They target health promotion, well-being and social integration, in order to counteract 'learned helplessness' since people with suspected dementia may be particularly vulnerable to this (Flannery 2002). Learned helplessness is a psychological state that is associated with mood disorders and results when a person who is unable to control one situation incorrectly assumes that she or he is unable to exercise reasonable control in other situations as well.

There is a fourth step in the framework for reducing excess disability in early dementia. This provides psychological treatment for people and their carers who are depressed or anxious, but is out of the scope of the present chapter since in this primary care-based memory clinic low estimates of 14 per cent for anxiety and 2 per cent for depression were noted, probably because early recognition practices by local GPs were well established (Moniz-Cook *et al.* 2001a, 2001b). In contrast, Clare *et al.* (2002) report higher levels in recently diagnosed memory clinic attendees, with 40 per cent experiencing anxiety and 17 per cent depression. Where people with dementia and their families have developed learned helplessness and/or mood disorders, psychological therapies such as cognitive behavioural therapy, relaxation strategies offered individually (Balasubramanyam, Stanley and Kunik 2007; Flannery 2002; James 2002; Scholey and Woods 2003; Suhr, Anderson and Tranel 1999; Walker 2004) or in groups (Kipling, Bailey and Charlesworth 1999), interpersonal therapy (James, Postma and Mackenzie 2003) and group psychotherapy (Chapter 9) have all been used with some success to alleviate anxiety and depression. There has been one randomised controlled trial of brief psychodynamic interpersonal therapy which reported no evidence to support the widespread introduction of brief psychotherapy in early dementia (Burns *et al.* 2005). Anxious or depressed carers have also benefited from psychological treatments (Marriott *et al.* 2000).

As was seen in some case studies above, delivering timely psychosocial intervention in early dementia or where a dementia diagnosis is not yet evident is not straightforward. Engagement in intervention often depends on the attitudes, beliefs and aspirations of the person, their spouse or partner and their wider family or support systems. Where differing attitudes, beliefs and aspirations or tensions exist, psycho-educational family conferences (Woolford 1998) may help, or separate practitioners may be required to meet the aspirations of the person with dementia and of the carer. However, for most families, the studies described in this chapter and related interventions in North America suggest that it is possible for skilled practitioners to offer prophylactic psychosocial intervention within a longitudinal tracking system (see, for example, Callahan *et al.* 2006; Mittelman *et al.* 2006; Teri *et al.* 2005).

References

Balasubramanyam, V., Stanley, M. and Kunik, M. (2007) 'Cognitive behavioural therapy for anxiety in dementia.' *Dementia* 6, 299–307.
Bowler, J. and Hachinski, V. (eds) (2003) *Vascular Cognitive Impairment: Preventable Dementia.* Oxford: Oxford University Press.

Brenes, G., Guralnik, J., Williamson, J., Frief, L., *et al.* (2005) 'The influence of anxiety on the progression of disability.' *Journal of the American Society of Geriatric Medicine 53*, 34–39.

Burns, A., Gutherie, E., Marino-Francis, F., Busby, C., *et al.* (2005) 'Brief psychotherapy in Alzheimer's disease: randomised controlled trial.' *British Journal of Psychiatry 187*, 143–147.

Callahan, C., Boustani, M., Unverzagt, F., Austrom, M., *et al.* (2006) 'Effectiveness of collaborative care for older adults with Alzheimer's disease in primary care: a randomised controlled trial.' *Journal of the American Medical Association 295*, 2148–2157.

Camp, C., Bird, M. and Cherry, K. (2000) 'Retrieval Strategies as a Rehabilitation Aid for Cognitive Loss in Pathological Aging.' In R.D. Hill, L. Backman and A.S. Neely (eds) *Cognitive Rehabilitation in Old Age.* Oxford: Oxford University Press.

Carter, P. and Everitt, A. (1998) 'Conceptualising practice with older people: friendship and conversation.' *Ageing and Society 18*, 79–99.

Clare, L. (2008) *Neuropsychological Rehabilitation and People with Dementia.* Hove: Psychology Press.

Clare, L. and Woods, R.T. (eds) (2001) *Cognitive Rehabilitation in Dementia.* Hove: Psychology Press.

Clare, L., Wilson, B., Carter, G., Breen, K., Berrios, G. and Hodges, J. (2002) 'Depression and anxiety in memory clinic attendees and their carers: implications for evaluating the effectiveness of cognitive rehabilitation interventions.' *International Journal of Geriatric Psychiatry 17*, 962–967.

Eggermont, L. and Scherder, E. (2006) 'Physical activity in dementia: a review of the literature and implications for psychosocial intervention in primary care.' *Dementia 5*, 411–428.

Engelborghs, S., Vloeberghs, E., Maertens, K., Marien, P., *et al.* (2004) 'Correlations between cognitive, behavioural and psychological findings and levels of vitamin B_{12} and folate in patients with dementia.' *International Journal of Geriatric Psychiatry 19*, 365–370.

Finnema, E., Dröes, R.M., Ribble, M. and Van Tillberg, W. (2000) 'The effects of emotion-orientated approaches in the care for persons suffering from dementia: a review of the literature.' *International Journal of Geriatric Psychiatry 15*, 141–161.

Flannery, R. (2002) 'Treating learned helplessness in the elderly dementia patient: preliminary inquiry.' *American Journal of Alzheimer's Disease and Other Dementias 17*, 6, 345–349.

Gilliard, J., Means, R., Beattie, A. and Daker-White, G. (2005) 'Dementia care in England and the social model of disability: lessons and issues.' *Dementia 4*, 571–586.

Gitlin L., Corcoran, M., Winter, L., Boyce, A. and Marcus, S. (1999) 'Predicting participation and adherence to a home environmental intervention among family caregivers of persons with dementia.' *Family Relations 48*, 4, 363–372.

Grady, C. (2007) 'Cognitive Reserve in Healthy Ageing and Alzheimer's Disease: Evidence for Compensatory Organisation of Brain Networks.' In Y. Stern (ed.) *Cognitive Reserve: Theory and Applications.* New York, NY: Taylor and Francis.

Hill, R.D., Backman, L. and Neely, A.S. (eds) (2002) *Cognitive Rehabilitation in Old Age.* Oxford: Oxford University Press.

James, A. and Sabin, N. (2005) 'An evaluation of a memory remediation group: do carers benefit?' *PSIGE – Psychology Specialists Promoting Psychological Wellbeing in Late Life – Newsletter 91*, 22–27.

James, I. (2002) 'Treatment of Distress in People with Severe Dementia using Cognitive-behavioural Concepts.' In S. Benson (ed.) *Dementia Topics for the Millennium and Beyond.* London: Hawker Publications.

James, I., Postma, K. and Mackenzie, L. (2003) 'Using an IPT conceptualization to treat a depressed person with dementia.' *Behavioural and Cognitive Psychotherapy 31*, 451–456.

Jané-Llopis, E., Hosman, C., Jenkins, R. and Anderson, P. (2002) 'Predictors of efficacy in depression programmes: meta-analysis.' *British Journal of Psychiatry 183*, 384–397.

Kelly, K., Pickett, W., Yiannakoulias, N., Rowe, B., *et al.* (2003) 'Medication use and falls in community dwelling older persons.' *Age and Ageing 32*, 503–509.

Kipling, T., Bailey, M. and Charlesworth, G. (1999) 'The feasibility of a cognitive behavioural therapy group for men with mild/moderate cognitive impairment.' *Behavioural and Cognitive Psychotherapy 27*, 189–193.

Marriott, A., Donaldson, C., Tarrier, N. and Burns, A. (2000) 'Effectiveness of cognitive-behavioural family intervention in reducing the burden of care in carers of patients with Alzheimer's disease.' *British Journal of Psychiatry 176*, 557–562.

Mittelman, M., William, P., Haley, E., Clay, O. and Roth, D. (2006) 'Improving caregiver well-being delays nursing home placement of patients with Alzheimer disease.' *Neurology 67*, 1592–1599.

Moniz-Cook, E.D. (2008) 'Assessment and Psychosocial Intervention for Older People with Suspected Dementia: A Memory Clinic Perspective.' In K. Laidlaw and B. Knight (eds) *Handbook of Emotional Disorders in Late Life: Assessment and Treatment.* Oxford: Oxford University Press.

Moniz-Cook, E., Gibson, G. and Win, T. (1997) 'Memory clinics in general practice in Hull: is there a role for crisis prevention and early psychosocial practice?' *PSIGE – Psychology Specialists Promoting Psychological Wellbeing in Late Life – Newsletter 60*, 15–20.

Moniz-Cook, E., Gibson, G., Win, T., Agar, S. and Wang, M. (1998) 'A preliminary study of the effects of early intervention with people with dementia and their families in a memory clinic.' *Aging and Mental Health 2*, 166–175.

Moniz-Cook, E., Wang, M., Campion, P., Gardiner, E., *et al.* (2001a) 'Early psychosocial intervention through a memory clinic – a randomised controlled trial.' *Gerontology 47*, 526.

Moniz-Cook, E., Campion, P., Wang, M., *et al.* (2001b) 'Early psychosocial intervention through a memory clinic: a randomised controlled trial (PCC1040).' *The Research Findings Register.* Summary number 541 (www.controlled-trials.com/mrct/trials/%7C/1053/31809.html, accessed 6 August 2008).

Moniz-Cook, E.D., Manthorpe, J., Carr, I., Gibson, G. and Vernooij-Dassen, M. (2006) 'Facing the future: a qualitative study of older people referred to a memory clinic prior to assessment and diagnosis.' *Dementia 5*, 375–395.

Moniz-Cook, E.D., Elston, C., Gardiner, E., Agar, S., *et al.* (2008) 'Can training community mental health nurses to support family carers reduce behavioural problems in dementia? An exploratory pragmatic randomised controlled trial.' *International Journal of Geriatric Psychiatry 23*, 185–191.

Naidoo, J. and Willis, J. (2000) *Health Promotion: Foundations for Practice.* London: Ballière Tindall.

Nutbeam, D. (1998) 'Comprehensive strategies for health promotion for older people: past lessons and future opportunities.' *Australasian Journal on Ageing 17*, 3, 120–127.

Oliver, D., Daly, F., Martin, F. and McMurdo, M. (2004) 'Risk factors and risk assessment tools for falls in hospital in-patients: a systematic review.' *Age and Ageing 33*, 122–130.

Orani, M., Moniz-Cook, E.D., Binetti, G., Zaneri, G., *et al.* (2003) 'An electronic memory aid to support prospective memory in patients in the early stages of Alzheimer's disease.' *Aging and Mental Health 7*, 22–27.

Pinquart. M. (2002) 'Creating and maintaining purpose in life in old age: a meta-analysis.' *Ageing International 27*, 2, 90–114.

Purandare, N., Ballard, C. and Burns, A. (2005) 'Preventing dementia.' *Advances in Psychiatric Treatment 11*, 176–183.

Richards, K., Moniz-Cook E.D., Duggan, P., Carr, I. and Wang, M. (2003) 'Defining "early dementia" and monitoring intervention: what measures are useful in family caregiving?' *Aging and Mental Health 7*, 7–14.

Russell, V., Proctor, L. and Moniz-Cook, E.D. (1989) 'The influence of a relative support group on carers' emotional distress.' *Journal of Advanced Nursing 14*, 863–867.

Sabat, S. (1994) 'Excess disability and malignant social psychology: a case study of Alzheimer's disease.' *Journal of Community and Applied Social Psychology 4*, 157–66.

Sacks, O. (1970) *The Man Who Mistook His Wife for a Hat.* New York, NY: Simon and Schuster.

Scholey, K. and Woods, B. (2003) 'A series of brief cognitive therapy interventions of people experiencing both dementia and depression: a description of techniques and common themes.' *Clinical Psychology and Psychotherapy 10*, 175–185.

Spector, A., Thorgrimsen, L., Woods, R.T., Royan, L., *et al.* (2003) 'Efficacy of an evidence-based cognitive stimulation therapy programme for people with dementia: randomised controlled trial.' *British Journal of Psychiatry 183*, 248–254.

Suhr, J., Anderson, S. and Tranel, D. (1999) 'Progressive muscle relaxation in the management of behavioural disturbance in Alzheimer's disease.' *Neuropsychological Rehabilitation 9*, 31–44.

Takahashi, K., Tamura, J. and Tokoro, M. (1997) 'Patterns of social relationships and well-being among the elderly.' *International Journal of Behavioural Development 21*, 417–430.

Teri, L. and Truax, P. (1994) 'Assessment of depression in dementia patients: associations of care mood with depression ratings.' *Gerontologist 34*, 231–234.

Teri, L., Logsdon, R., Uomoto, J. and McCurry, S. (1997) 'Behavioural treatment of depression in dementia patients: a controlled clinical trial.' *Journals of Gerontology B: Psychological Sciences and Social Sciences 52B*, 159–166.

Teri, L., Logsdon, R.G. and McCurry, S.M. (2002) 'Nonpharmacologic treatment of behavioural disturbance in dementia.' *The Medical Clinics of North America 86*, 641–656.

Teri, L., McCurry, S.M., Logsdon, R. and Gibbons, L.E. (2005) 'Training community consultants to help family members improve dementia care.' *Gerontologist 45*, 802–811.

Tuokko, H.A. and Hultsch, D.F. (eds) (2006) *Mild Cognitive Impairment: International Perspectives.* New York, NY: Taylor and Francis.

Walker, D.A. (2004) 'Cognitive behavioural therapy for depression in a person with Alzheimer's dementia.' *Behavioural and Cognitive Psychotherapy 32*, 495–550.

Woods, R.T. and Clare, L. (2008) 'Psychological Intervention and Dementia'. In R.T. Woods and L. Clare (eds) *Handbook of the Clinical Psychology of Ageing*, 2nd edn. Chichester: Wiley.

Woolford, H. (1998) 'An intervention to assist dementia care: the psycho-educational family conference.' *PSIGE – Psychology Specialists Promoting Psychological Wellbeing in Late Life – Newsletter 65*, 32–34.

Zarit, S.H., Zarit, J.M. and Reever, K.E. (1982) 'Memory training for severe memory loss: effects on senile dementia patients and their families.' *Gerontologist 22*, 373–377.

PART II

Cognitive and Memory Support

Chapter 4

Working with Memory Problems

Cognitive Rehabilitation in Early Dementia

Linda Clare

Overview

Memory problems are an important part of the changes experienced by the majority of people who are in the early stages of dementia (Brandt and Rich 1995), and the development of memory problems can have a profound impact on sense of self, daily life and relationships. The person with a memory problem may feel angry or distressed, or fear he or she is 'going mad'. Families, friends and supporters may experience frustration or irritation, and often find it hard to know how to respond. Helping with memory problems, therefore, has the potential to enable the person with dementia to feel more in control, and to assist others in responding appropriately. For this reason, targeting memory-related concerns is likely to be an important part of early intervention in dementia (Clare *et al.* 1999). This chapter will outline what is meant by cognitive rehabilitation, give some examples of specific techniques, and consider what factors are important when trying to implement a cognitive rehabilitation approach.

Cognitive rehabilitation

A useful framework for helping with memory and other cognitive problems is provided by the cognitive rehabilitation approach. This model was initially developed through work with younger brain-injured people, and more recently it has been applied to address the needs of people with dementia (Clare and Woods 2001). It has been defined as: 'any intervention strategy or technique which intends to enable clients or patients, and their families, to live with, manage, by-pass, reduce or come to terms with deficits precipitated by injury to the brain' (Wilson 1997, p.487).

Within this framework, the memory problems of early dementia can be tackled in two main ways (Clare and Wilson 1997):

- building on remaining memory skills

- finding ways of compensating for impaired aspects of memory.

Rehabilitation is conducted in the context of a natural trajectory of change over time, which varies according to the individual, the nature of the impairment, and the social context (Clare and Woods 2004). Due to the progressive nature of Alzheimer's disease, rehabilitation goals will change over time in a way that reflects this trajectory (Clare 2003). In the early stages of dementia, changes in cognitive functioning and the impact of these on daily life and relationships are likely to form a major focus, so cognitive rehabilitation may be particularly relevant. Although people with early dementia may have some obvious and severe memory problems, they are to some extent still able to learn some new information, retain information they have learned, improve their practical skills, and adapt or change their behaviour (see, for example, Camp *et al.* 1993; Little *et al.* 1986). This is because in the early stages of dementia different aspects of memory are affected to different degrees (Brandt and Rich 1995), and some are not affected at all. Memory for recent events and personal experiences is likely to be most severely affected, while the ability to carry out practical skills is least affected. Although taking in new information can be very difficult, established memories tend to be retained reasonably well (Christensen *et al.* 1998). This means that if the right kind of help is given, some improvements in memory and everyday functioning may be possible (Bäckman 1992). Specific techniques have been described that are suitable for use with people who have dementia, whether the aim is to build on remaining memory or to compensate for memory losses.

Building on remaining memory

Building on remaining memory can involve either aspects of memory that are impaired or aspects of memory that are relatively intact. Helping people take in information depends on using the impaired aspects of memory. Methods which may be helpful include the following:

- *Elaborating on the information that needs to be remembered* (Bird and Luszcz 1993). This can be done by linking it to other knowledge. For example, the name Butler can be linked to the job done by a butler. The role of a butler could be play acted as well, since involving multiple senses can aid learning (Karlsson *et al.* 1989).

- *Mnemonics.* These can sometimes help with remembering names (Hill *et al.* 1987). A prominent feature of the person's face or appearance is identified and linked with the sound of the first letter of their name. For example, Rab Butler, whose photograph taken in late middle age shows a balding head, might be remembered as 'rather bald' Rab Butler.

- *Expanding rehearsal.* This is sometimes referred to as spaced retrieval (Brush and Camp 1998; Camp and Stevens 1990). After the information has been given to the person with dementia, questions are asked at gradually increasing intervals to elicit the information. The first interval might be as little as 20 or 30 seconds, the second interval is double the length of the first, and the process continues until the desired retention interval is reached. If the information is not recalled, the intervals are halved until the person can recall it again. For example, having learned the name Rab Butler in the ways described above, the person could be asked to recall the name after intervals of 30 seconds, one minute, two minutes, and so on.

- *Errorless learning.* It may be helpful to try to reduce the risk of the person making mistakes while learning (Clare *et al.* 1999, 2000, 2001). This means that guessing should be discouraged. If the person is unsure, the correct information can be supplied, rather than risking a wrong guess.

Building on the more preserved aspects of memory generally involves rehearsal and practice of activities of daily living and other skills (Josephsson *et al.* 1993; Zanetti *et al.* 1994). Practice is structured in such a way that the person is guided through the activities by means of prompts and cues, rather than having to recall what needs to be done. The prompts and cues, which may be verbal, gestural, pictorial or written, can be withdrawn gradually as the routines become more established. This kind of approach may be particularly important for maintaining independence.

Case example – Alan

Alan was frustrated and upset because he could not remember the names of the other members of his social club. To help him learn the names, photographs were taken of the club members and the names were practised one at a time. For each name, Alan thought of a mnemonic (for example, Caroline with the curl), and expanding rehearsal was used to help him recall the name over a 20-minute interval. Later, Alan took the photographs to the club and tried matching them to the members and then recalling their names. By doing this, and practising with the photographs each day, Alan managed to learn all the names. He continued to practise, and still recalled all the names perfectly a year later (taken from Clare et al. 1999).

Compensating for memory problems

If information cannot be held in memory, it may be possible to compensate for this by providing access to it in alternative ways. Memory aids may take over some of the functions of memory. For example, a calendar or diary can be used to find out the date (Hanley 1986), while a memory book or memory wallet containing important personal information can give reminders about things to say in conversation with others (Bourgeois 1990, 1992). Cues can be built into the person's surroundings. For example, signs on drawers and cupboards can indicate where things are kept, while checklists can describe how to carry out practical tasks.

In order for the person with dementia to make use of memory aids and environmental adaptations, he or she needs to understand exactly what they are for (Woods 1996a) and develop the habit or routine of using them. This can be done by prompting the person to use them regularly and providing cues to make sure this is successful. As the routine becomes established, the cues and prompts can be gradually reduced.

Case example – Evelyn

Evelyn often asked her husband Eric 'What day is it today?' Eric had bought Evelyn a calendar that showed one day to a page, but grumbled that she had never used it. Eric agreed to prompt Evelyn to look at her calendar and tell him the day every morning, afternoon and evening. Each time Evelyn asked him what day it was, he also suggested that she look at her calendar. After a few weeks, Evelyn was using the calendar regularly and Eric gradually stopped prompting her. Both Evelyn and Eric felt much happier now that Evelyn was using the calendar instead of asking Eric the same question repeatedly (taken from Clare et al. 2000).

Implementing cognitive rehabilitation

Cognitive rehabilitation interventions for people with dementia may be carried out individually (Clare *et al.* 1999), with families (Quayhagen and Quayhagen 1989), in a group (Sandman 1993), or as part of a wider programme of psychosocial intervention (Moniz-Cook *et al.* 1998) or 'elder rehab' (Arkin 1996). The interventions may be delivered primarily by health professionals, carers, friends or volunteers. Whichever method is chosen, and whoever is involved in carrying them out, it is essential to ensure that the intervention is sensitive to individual needs. It is also important to acknowledge that some people with early stage dementia will prefer not to address their memory problems in this way, and their choice must be respected. If appropriate, advice may still be given to carers or family members on responding to memory difficulties. Guidelines on implementing cognitive rehabilitation interventions are provided by Bäckman (1992), Clare *et al.* (1999), and Woods (1996b). These suggest that cognitive rehabilitation interventions should be:

- directed at specific individual goals which are realistic, practically relevant and meaningful to the person

- based on an assessment of the individual's strengths and difficulties in memory and other areas of cognitive functioning, including an observation of functioning in relevant real-life settings

- founded on a shared understanding of the aims and goals of the intervention and the methods used

- sensitive to the emotional impact of memory problems and the wider needs of people and families adjusting to the onset of dementia

- carried out in a collaborative manner involving not only the person with dementia but also his or her family members or supporters, who may be crucial to the success of any intervention and are in a position to integrate the methods of cognitive rehabilitation into daily life

- sufficiently extensive to facilitate change, with ongoing input after the end of the main intervention to allow gains to be maintained.

Following these guidelines may help to ensure that the needs of the person with dementia are met at each stage of the process of working together to tackle the memory problems.

Conclusion

Memory problems signalling the onset of dementia can be frightening, upsetting and frustrating. The work described in this chapter shows that although the memory problems cannot be cured, there are some things that can help. However, it should be noted that there is a lack of randomised controlled trials of individualised cognitive rehabilitation for people with early stage dementia, highlighting the need for more evidence to support the use of such interventions (Clare *et al.* 2003). A review of the existing research on memory therapy concluded that it was a 'probably efficacious' method of helping people with dementia (Gatz *et al.* 1998). Interventions of this kind, provided they are implemented in a sensitive manner, may assist individuals and families and improve aspects of their daily lives.

References

Arkin, S.M. (1996) 'Volunteers in partnership: an Alzheimer's rehabilitation program delivered by students.' *The American Journal of Alzheimer's Disease 11*, 12–22.

Bäckman, L. (1992) 'Memory training and memory improvement in Alzheimer's disease: rules and exceptions.' *Acta Neurologica Scandinavica, Supplement 139*, 84–89.

Bird, M. and Luszcz, M. (1993) 'Enhancing memory performance in Alzheimer's disease: acquisition assistance and cue effectiveness.' *Journal of Clinical and Experimental Neuropsychology 15*, 921–932.

Bourgeois, M.S. (1990) 'Enhancing conversation skills in patients with Alzheimer's disease using a prosthetic memory aid.' *Journal of Applied Behavior Analysis 23*, 29–42.

Bourgeois, M.S. (1992) 'Evaluating memory wallets in conversations with persons with dementia.' *Journal of Speech and Hearing Research 35*, 1344–1357.

Brandt, J. and Rich, J.B. (1995) 'Memory Disorders in the Dementias.' In A.D. Baddeley, B.A. Wilson and F.N. Watts (eds) *Handbook of Memory Disorders.* Chichester: Wiley.

Brush, J.A. and Camp, C.J. (1998) *A Therapy Technique for Improving Memory: Spaced Retrieval.* Beechwood, OH: Myers Research Institute, Menorah Park Center for the Aging.

Camp, C.J. and Stevens, A.B. (1990) 'Spaced retrieval: a memory intervention for dementia of the Alzheimer's type (DAT).' *Clinical Gerontologist 10*, 58–61.

Camp, C.J., Foss, J.W., Stevens, A.B., Reichard, C.C., McKitrick, L.A. and O'Hanlon, A.M. (1993) 'Memory training in normal and demented elderly populations: the E-I-E-I-O model.' *Experimental Aging Research 19*, 277–290.

Christensen, H., Kopelman, M.D., Stanhop, N., Lorentz, L. and Owen, P. (1998) 'Rates of forgetting in Alzheimer dementia.' *Neuropsychologia 36*, 547–557.

Clare, L. (2003) 'Rehabilitation for People with Dementia.' In B.A. Wilson (ed.) *Neuropsychological Rehabilitation: Theory and Practice.* Lisse: Swets & Zeitlinger.

Clare, L. and Wilson, B.A. (1997) *Coping with Memory Problems: A Practical Guide for People with Memory Impairments and their Relatives and Friends.* Bury St Edmunds: Thames Valley Test Company.

Clare, L. and Woods, R.T. (2001) *Cognitive Rehabilitation in Dementia.* Hove: Psychology Press.

Clare, L. and Woods, R.T. (2004) 'Cognitive training and cognitive rehabilitation for people with early-stage Alzheimer's disease: A review.' *Neuropsychological Rehabilitation 14*, 385–401.

Clare, L., Wilson, B.A., Breen, K. and Hodges, J.R. (1999) 'Errorless learning of face–name associations in early Alzheimer's disease.' *Neurocase 5*, 37–46.

Clare, L., Wilson, B.A., Carter, G., Gosses, A., Breen, K. and Hodges, J.R. (2000) 'Intervening with everyday memory problems in early Alzheimer's disease: an errorless learning approach.' *Journal of Clinical and Experimental Neuropsychology 22*, 132–146.

Clare, L., Wilson, B.A., Carter, G., Hodges, J.R. and Adams, M. (2001) 'Long-term maintenance of treatment gains following a cognitive rehabilitation in early dementia of Alzheimer type: a single case study.' *Neuropsychological Rehabilitation. Special Issue: Cognitive Rehabilitation in Dementia 11*, 477–494.

Clare, L., Woods, B., Moniz-Cook, E., Orrell, M. and Spector, A. (2003) 'Cognitive rehabilitation and cognitive training interventions targeting memory functioning in early stage Alzheimer's disease and vascular dementia (review).' In *The Cochrane Database of Systematic Reviews*, Issue 4. Chichester: Wiley.

Gatz, M., Fiske, A., Fox, L., Kaskie, B., Kasl-Godley, J., McCallum, T. and Wetherell, J.L. (1998) 'Empirically validated psychological treatments for older adults.' *Journal of Mental Health and Aging* 4, 9–45.

Hanley, I. (1986) 'Reality Orientation in the Care of the Elderly Patient with Dementia – Three Case Studies.' In I. Hanley and M. Gilhooly (eds) *Psychological Therapies for the Elderly*. Beckenham: Croom Helm.

Hill, R.D., Evankovich, K.D., Sheikh, J.I. and Yesavage, J.A. (1987) 'Imagery mnemonic training in a patient with primary degenerative dementia.' *Psychology and Aging* 2, 204–205.

Josephsson, S., Bäckman, L., Borell, L., Bernspang, B., Nygard, L. and Ronnberg, L. (1993) 'Supporting everyday activities in dementia: an intervention study.' *International Journal of Geriatric Psychiatry* 8, 395–400.

Karlsson, T., Bäckman, L., Herlitz, A., Nilsson, L., Winblad, B. and Osterlind, P. (1989) 'Memory improvement at different stages of Alzheimer's disease.' *Neuropsychologia* 27, 737–742.

Little, A.G., Volans, P.J., Hemsley, D.R. and Levy, R. (1986) 'The retention of new information in senile dementia.' *British Journal of Clinical Psychology* 25, 71–72.

Moniz-Cook, E., Agar, S., Gibson, G., Win, T. and Wang, M. (1998) 'A preliminary study of the effects of early intervention with people with dementia and their families in a memory clinic.' *Aging and Mental Health* 2, 199–211.

Quayhagen, M.P. and Quayhagen, M. (1989) 'Differential effects of family-based strategies on Alzheimer's disease.' *Gerontologist* 29, 150–155.

Sandman, C.A. (1993) 'Memory rehabilitation in Alzheimer's disease: preliminary findings.' *Clinical Gerontologist* 13, 19–33.

Wilson, B.A. (1997) 'Cognitive rehabilitation: how it is and how it might be.' *Journal of the International Neuropsychological Society* 3, 487–496.

Woods, R.T. (1996a) 'Cognitive Approaches to the Management of Dementia.' In R.G. Morris (ed.) *The Cognitive Neuropsychology of Alzheimer-type Dementia*. Oxford: Oxford University Press.

Woods, R.T. (1996b) 'Psychological "Therapies" in Dementia.' In R.T. Woods (ed.) *Handbook of the Clinical Psychology of Ageing*. Chichester: Wiley.

Zanetti, O., Magni, E., Binetti, G., Bianchetti, A. and Trabucchi, M. (1994) 'Is procedural memory stimulation effective in Alzheimer's disease?' *International Journal of Geriatric Psychiatry* 9, 1006–1007.

Further Reading and related references

Clare, L. (2002) 'We'll fight it as long as we can: coping with the onset of Alzheimer's disease.' *Aging and Mental Health* 6, 139–148.

Clare, L. (2003) 'Cognitive training and cognitive rehabilitation for people with early-stage dementia.' *Reviews in Clinical Gerontology* 13, 75–83.

Clare, L. (2003) 'Managing threats to self: awareness in early-stage Alzheimer's disease.' *Social Science and Medicine* 57, 1017–1029.

Clare, L. (2004) 'Assessment and Intervention in Dementia of Alzheimer Type.' In A.D. Baddeley, B.A. Wilson and M. Kopelman (eds) *The Essential Handbook of Memory Disorders for Clinicians*. Chichester: Wiley.

Clare, L. (2004) 'Cognitive Rehabilitation for People with Early-stage Dementia.' In M.T. Marshall (ed.) *Perspectives on Rehabilitation and Dementia*. London: Jessica Kingsley Publishers.

Clare, L. (2005) 'Cognitive Rehabilitation in Early-stage Dementia: Evidence, Practice and Future Directions.' In P. Halligan and D. Wade (eds) *Evidence for the Effectiveness of Cognitive Rehabilitation*. Oxford: Oxford University Press.

Clare, L. and Cox, S. (2003) 'Improving service approaches and outcomes for people with complex needs through consultation and involvement.' *Disability and Society* 18, 935–953.

Clare, L., Baddeley, A., Moniz-Cook, E.D. and Woods, R.T. (2003) 'A quiet revolution: advances in the understanding of dementia.' *The Psychologist* 16, 250–254.

Clare, L., Wilson, B.A., Carter, G., Roth, I. and Hodges, J.R. (2002) 'Relearning of face–name associations in early-stage Alzheimer's disease.' *Neuropsychology* 16, 538–547.

Clare, L., Wilson, B.A., Carter, G., Roth, I. and Hodges, J.R. (2002) 'Assessing awareness in early-stage Alzheimer's disease: development and piloting of the Memory Awareness Rating Scale.' *Neuropsychological Rehabilitation* 12, 341–362.

Clare, L., Wilson, B.A., Carter, G., Breen, K., Berrios, G.E. and Hodges, J.R. (2002) 'Depression and anxiety in memory clinic attenders and their carers: implications for evaluating the effectiveness of cognitive rehabilitation interventions.' *International Journal of Geriatric Psychiatry* 17, 962–967.

Clare, L., Wilson, B.A., Carter, G. and Hodges, J.R. (2003) 'Cognitive rehabilitation as a component of early intervention in dementia: a single case study.' *Aging and Mental Health 7*, 15–21.

Clare, L., Wilson, B.A., Carter, G., Roth, I. and Hodges, J.R. (2004) 'Awareness in early-stage Alzheimer's disease: relationship to outcome of cognitive rehabilitation.' *Journal of Clinical and Experimental Neuropsychology 26*, 215–226.

Chapter 5

Cognitive Stimulation for People with Mild Cognitive Impairment and Early Dementia

Inge Cantegreil-Kallen, Jocelyne de Rotrou
and Anne-Sophie Rigaud

Overview

Cognitive Stimulation (CS) was developed for people with early dementia at Hôpital Broca in France. In the late 1990s it acted as the evidence base for reality orientation in dementia, reflected in the now withdrawn Cochrane review (Spector *et al.* 1998). The aim of CS is to slow down the rate of overall cognitive decline by using a functional approach that concentrates on reinforcing the cognitive 'reserve' capacity. CS has been used with people in early and moderate stages of dementia. In this chapter research into cognitive stimulation in France is outlined and an example of the contents of a cognitive stimulation session is also described. The chapter then focuses on CS as a therapeutic intervention in early dementia, since learning specific cognitive strategies is a valuable way in which to delay the onset of problems. Moreover, it is suggested that CS for people with Mild Cognitive Impairment (MCI) can, by virtue of its goals, methods and framework, help to differentiate between those whose condition is 'stable' and those considered 'at risk' of developing dementia.

The concept: definition, goals and methods

Cognitive Stimulation (CS), where parts of the brain can take over the functions of other parts that may be damaged, is based on the notion of cerebral plasticity. It aims to optimise cognitive function using a range of mental activities. These make up the treatment of memory-related concerns associated with both normal ageing as well as conditions such as dementia. It can be described as a global approach (see Clare and Woods 2004) that is concerned with both cognitive factors (such as attention/concentration, orientation, different types of memory, visual-constructive abilities, executive function, and verbal fluency) and psychosocial factors, such as self-confidence, motivation, socialisation, and affective states.

Cognitive Stimulation programmes are varied and often require adapting to the target population, or to achieve the desired outcome. Programmes in France exist for older people who complain of memory difficulties, yet perform adequately on neuropsychological screening tests, and thus remain within designated norms as well as people who may have Mild Cognitive Impairment, i.e. those whose test performance falls slightly below the established norm and people who present with Alzheimer-type dementia.

For older people who complain of memory loss while demonstrating normal cognitive ability, CS offers a programme of reassurance for concerns associated with memory difficulties, and thus enhances self-confidence through acquisition or relearning of recall strategies. Offering stimulation for complaints of memory difficulties in the absence of objective decline may prevent disability, since memory difficulties can precede cognitive deterioration.

CS programmes in France were developed in the early 1980s aimed primarily at people with Alzheimer's disease. Jocelyne de Rotrou developed a neuropedagogical treatment for people in the early stages of Alzheimer's disease, whilst working in the Department of Clinical Gerontology at Broca Hospital in Paris. Rotrou took her inspiration from the findings of neuropedagogy, primarily practised in the United States, where the underlying hypothesis is that people with Alzheimer's disease can have capacity for cognitive storage, and that this albeit limited capacity can be stimulated. It is suggested that this cognitive 'reserve capacity' may allow the person with dementia to benefit, to some extent, from cueing and memory strategies. In Alzheimer's disease, implicit memory, which is typically preserved for a longer period than episodic memory, can also respond to regular stimulation. Therefore, offering people with dementia a set of exercises that takes reserve capacity into account allows them to maintain, for a period of time, a better level of cognitive performance than that of equivalent people with dementia who do not receive cognitive stimulation. The goals of CS are twofold:

1. To preserve cognitive function for as long as possible, and thus delay the loss of abilities and enhance performance of everyday living activities, i.e. the ultimate goal being the preservation of a person's independence.

2. To increase or re-establish self-worth by improving self-confidence and providing motivation to perform activities that require cognitive effort.

The methods used in CS are designed to achieve these goals. Exercises are designed to stimulate the various areas of cognition: memory, concentration, language, executive function, spatio-temporal orientation and visuo-constructive abilities. The person with dementia applies strategies based on mental imagery, categorical classification and semantic (word) association, with the aim of preserving and even improving episodic and semantic memory, as well as consolidating implicit memory. The stimulation exercises are developed according to the preferred interests and activities of the older person and these are then grouped by theme. Each theme contains exercises of different types, focusing in turn on memory, concentration, language and executive abilities. CS thus offers an approach that incorporates the range of domains of cognitive activity. Based on the notion that a person's emotional state and cognitive functioning are interdependent, this global vision of therapy means that treatment is extended to the person's psychosocial functioning in a number of ways. First, motivation can play an important role in intellectual functioning. Second, cognitive and psycho-affective functions influence social circumstances for the person with dementia and this includes involvement in family activities, and participation and maintenance of social relationships. CS thus focuses on oral expression in a group setting and sessions are organised in groups of eight to ten people, led by a psychologist trained in cognitive stimulation techniques. Groups meet weekly for one and a half hours over a period of 12 weeks. This framework allows the person with dementia to meet others with similar difficulties and can help the person to reduce anxiety about his or her own situation. Table 5.1 presents an example of a Cognitive Stimulation session.

Table 5.1 Contents of a Cognitive Stimulation session		
Exercises	Objectives (cognitive and psychosocial)	Daily life application
Diary • Participants present themselves and report what they have done in the past week.	• Reinforcing sense of identity and self-awareness. • Reinforcing episodic memory. • Reduction of apathy.	• Active participation in family and social life.
Newspaper review • Participants report on current (national and international) political, economical, social, cultural, news and sport events.	• Reinforcing socialisation (increasing the feeling of participating in community life). • Reinforcing semantic memory and verbal fluency. • Reduction of social withdrawal.	• Facilitating oral expression and communication. • Increasing interest in social events and in what is going on in society. • Reinforcing the feeling of belonging to a group.
Temporal/spatial orientation • Date, day of the week, season, anniversaries, holidays. • Participants describe the route and modes of transport they take to get to the hospital (e.g. underground stations, bus routes, etc.). • Recall of address and telephone number of the hospital.	• Temporal and spatial reorientation. • Emphasising topographic memory. • Emphasising biographic memory.	• Preserving autonomy in finding locations (e.g. shops, post office, bank, etc.).

Semantic categorisation
• Reading of a text.
• Classification of ideas or significant words.
• Construction of associations of learned words with current issues or a particular theme.
• Contextual encoding (e.g. writing sentences using the just learned words in order to memorise them).
	• Exercising functional competences:
	  o naming
	  o verbal organisation
	  o imagination
	  o reinforcing implicit word learning.
		• Improving oral expression and writing.
		• Translating ideas into adequate verbal expression.
		• Finding synonyms.
		• Spontaneous decision making.
		• Implicit automatic information processing.

Recall • Immediate free recall. • Cued recall of the learned items.	• Applying strategies used at encoding.	• Spontaneously using strategies in everyday life situations.

Exercises	Objectives (cognitive and psychosocial)	Daily life application
Executive function (linked to memory exercises): • Problem-solving. • Arithmetic (e.g. mental arithmetic, calculation of distances). • Attention/concentration (looking for differences, errors in sequences of items). • Logical and abstract thinking.	Improvement of: • Mental control: inhibition of irrelevant information. • Judgement. • Planning. • Abstract and logical reasoning. • Mental flexibility. • Decision-making competence.	Daily life executive skills: • Preparing a dish, paying an invoice, understanding a 'direction for use'.
Delayed recall • Free or cued recall of the learned items.	• Applying strategies used at encoding. • Maintenance of employed strategy after interruption.	• Spontaneously using strategies in everyday life situations.
Homework • Instructions about exercises participants have to do at home. • Provide encouragement and motivation to read newspapers.	• Maintaining social involvement by current affairs.	• Stimulating interest and motivation for intellectual tasks.

Evidence for Cognitive Stimulation as a therapeutic method in France

Cognitive Stimulation programmes designed for different types of individual presentation have been evaluated. For example, one study with 61 participants with normal cognitive functioning who reported memory loss found that the CS group had a statistically significant improvement compared with a 'non-stimulation' group, ($p<0.05$) on an associative memory test, i.e. the strongest measure of the wide-ranging strategies developed in the Cognitive Stimulation programme (Cimétière 1997). A study of the psychosocial benefits of CS with 124 'normal functioning' participants who reported memory loss (de Rotrou, Cantegreil-Kallen and Cimétière 2000), found a significant improvement ($p<0.05$) on two items of a self-evaluation scale of well-being (i.e. the importance that the person gave to his or her role in society, and the amount of interest he or she displayed in current events). Cognitive Stimulation did not impact on most other functions apart from two items relating to memory (i.e. remembering where certain objects were placed, and remembering a shopping list) where a statistically significant improvement was observed in individuals who had been stimulated (de Rotrou *et al.* 2000).

The CS programme designed for people with Alzheimer's disease has been evaluated by several control studies. The double-blind randomised controlled trial (Breuil *et al.* 1994) was seen as a key study for the evidence base of reality orientation in dementia in Spector and her colleagues' meta-analysis of the success of therapy based on reality orientation in people with dementia (Spector *et al.* 1998). The study consisted of 56 patients who were living at home, and demonstrated clear cognitive improvement in favour of the CS group, with statistically significant outcomes on episodic memory (p<0.01), and in particular on the recall of a list of words (p<0.009), as well as on spatio-temporal orientation. No differences between groups were noted on fluency tests and overall changes in cognition were not accompanied by improvements in activities of daily living or in behaviour. Another controlled study of 82 people with severe Alzheimer's disease living in a home facility showed a significant improvement (p<0.01) on the MMSE (two points) in favour of the stimulated group and a trend towards fewer day-to-day problems (Vidal *et al.* 1998).

Gosselin and colleagues evaluated the effectiveness of Cognitive Stimulation on behavioural outcomes by incorporating Cognitive Stimulation into a daily treatment programme for 29 institutionalised participants with severe Alzheimer's disease (Gosselin *et al.* 2003). They noted significant improvements in appetite and eating behaviour with associated reduction in distress among staff who were helping people at mealtimes.

New directions for Cognitive Stimulation in Mild Cognitive Impairment

MCI is a state that is thought by some to precede a diagnosis of dementia, since the person presents with reduced mnemonic (memory) or cognitive abilities, which do not impact on daily activities or meet the criteria for dementia. The concept of MCI is still in its infancy, but criteria include performance at 1.5 standard deviations below the age-scaled mean on neuropsychological tests, a Clinical Dementia Rating (CDR) score of <0.5 or a Global Deterioration Scale (GDS) of <3.0. Although people with MCI are considered to be an 'at risk' population, only a proportion go on to develop dementia, with the most frequently quoted statistics issued by the Mayo Clinic as 15 to 20 per cent each year (Petersen *et al.* 1999), although figures of 50 per cent progression in three to four years (Cameron and Clare 2004) and 31 per cent in three years (Zanetti *et al.* 2006) have been quoted. Identifying people with MCI who are 'at risk' of developing dementia is not easy, since the term reflects a heterogeneous condition of subsets where memory problem MCI is seen as the pre-clinical stage of Alzheimer's disease and multiple impaired cognitive problems associated with vascular dementia or MCI-VaD (Zanetti *et al.* 2006). Amnestic-MCI refers to deficits of memory and is associated with Alzheimer's disease, since the hippocampus and related temporal medial lobe structures which are associated with memory function are also seen as the initial sites of neurodegeneration in Alzheimer's disease. MCI is associated with deficits in the executive system (Zanetti *et al*. 2006). Deficits can be seen in problem solving, abstract thinking, attention, loss of mental flexibility, response inhibition and visuospatial tasks, all of which are associated with the frontal lobe (Albert 2002).

CS can contribute to research and a better understanding of MCI as a pre-clinical dementia state (Cantegreil-Kallen *et al*. 2002) in two ways: first, by exploring the potential of CS acting on cognitive reserve capacity to reduce the risk of progressing to dementia; second, to enhance the predictive value of early detection of Alzheimer's disease in MCI. The aim of the former would be to slow down the rate of overall cognitive decline and possibly delay the onset of disabling symptoms based on the notion that reserve capacity and plasticity of the human brain account for variability in the performance of cognitive activities. Since the risk of dementia is significantly increased among people with clear cognitive impairment beyond memory loss (Bozoki *et al*. 2001), i.e. they show more global cognitive impairment and exhibit episodic mnemonic deficits, there may be benefit in exploring the potential of CS in delaying the onset of dementia. CS involves practice at encoding and retrieval requiring some intact learning resources or reserve capacity. Early detection of dementia and subtypes is hypothetically possible within longitudinal studies, since lack of response to Cognitive Stimulation as measured by fine grained neuropsychological testing in memory, language, visuospatial ability and the range of executive functions may offer predictive potential. However, whilst there are neuropsychological tests of adequate sensitivity for early memory loss, e.g. the Profile of Cognitive Efficiency test (de Rotrou *et al*. 1991), measures of subtle changes in the executive functioning remain elusive.

Developing a CS programme for people with MCI

The benefits of CS are both the overall framework of the programme and the content of the specific exercises. The framework consists of weekly sessions with a psychologist who observes performances in terms of both the cognitive procedures used by the person and the contribution of the person's affective state on performance. Thus, the manner in which the person processes, learns and recalls information can provide information on the nature of the underlying deficit. The 12-week programme also allows observation of subtle functional and behavioural changes, since people with MCI present with an 'emotional vulnerability syndrome'. That is, they tend to visit their general practitioner more often than those who do not have MCI, suffer more frequently from (mild) depression and are significantly more vulnerable to stress or are dependent on their family and friends (Verhey and Visser 2000). In addition to within-session monitoring, the final outcome of a 12-week programme can also therefore be examined by particular neuropsychological subtests and self-report responses to questionnaires about affective state or mood.

The specific exercises that make up the programme are focused on four MCI cognitive characteristics that may or may not be of pre-clinical Alzheimer's disease (we refer to these as the 'at risk' MCI group), or may also serve to enhance cognitive reserve in those with MCI who do not progress to a dementia (referred to here as the 'stable' MCI group). These four MCI functional domains are diminished delayed recall, diminished category verbal fluency, diminished logical memory (i.e. paragraph recall) and diminished associative memory. Below we outline how particular cognitive exercises may help in the detection of early dementia or the delay of dementia through the maximising of cognitive reserve.

First, diminished delayed recall: this is the most common predictor of dementia and is also common in MCI, but free recall in episodic memory remains stable for three years, probably due to reserve capacity that allows use of compensatory strategies (Bäckman 2002). This may therefore be worthy of inclusion in a CS programme in MCI. Exercises targeting relearning and optimising of mnemonic strategies to enhance retrieval of acquired information may help those who do not go on to develop dementia (the 'stable' MCI subset) but those who progress to dementia (the 'at risk' subset) are unlikely to benefit. CS exercise performance on this task over time may add to the predictive value of CS in MCI and the detection of a developing early stage dementia, which in turn may allow opportunity for providing individual preventative cognitive and psychosocial support programmes to both subsets of people with MCI.

Second, diminished verbal fluency is the second most common deficit in early dementia (Palmer et al. 2002). Diminished fluency appears to be due to a reduced capacity to access the lexical stock (i.e. the capacity to identify strategies) as well as difficulty in applying strategies (Astell and Bucks 2002). People with MCI showing selective deficits in category fluency may therefore be at risk of developing Alzheimer's disease. Since category and letter fluency have different retrieval processes, neuropsychological responses in verbal learning and memory performance during Cognitive Stimulation exercises might act as potential markers for detecting those who may progress to developing Alzheimer's disease. Vocabulary exercises enrich the semantic stock as well as the relearning of strategies for recalling words or concepts, with the goal of improving the person's ability to compensate when unable to recall a word. A person's response following use of compensation strategies in CS can therefore act as a marker for 'at risk' of dementia in MCI and thus assist with early detection. Therapeutic potential is seen in that should the person fail to find a word, he or she would be able to locate a synonym or a description, thus reducing the fear of failure. This is particularly important since the anxiety of forgetting words during conversation can contribute to social withdrawal, and opportunity to improve efficacy early in the course of MCI may assist in preventing depression.

Third, diminished logical memory (paragraph recall) has been identified in people who are defined as having MCI with a Clinical Dementia Rating (CDR) score of <0.5 (Ferris 2002). Here CS exercises on text recall involve learning and repeating a paragraph or a very short story, where mnemonic strategies such as categorisation and the association of mental images play an important role in both detection (where 'stable' MCI and those 'at risk' of dementia can be differentiated) and memory improvement interventions.

Finally, diminished associative memory (i.e. the ability to learn associated words) is thought to differentiate those who remain stable from those who go on to develop dementia (Blackwell, Sahakian and Versey 2002). Pinpointing those who may be 'at risk' of dementia in a CS session may therefore be possible using observation of the degree to which the person is capable of benefiting from cueing, since this mechanism acts as an evaluative barometer for storage capacity, and the potential underlying disease process.

Conclusion and implications for future research

The evidence base for CS in maintaining cognition and psychological well-being in early stage dementia was developed in France (de Rotrou 2001; de Rotrou *et al.* 2002). It is now a recommended group treatment for people with mild to moderate dementia where treatment is offered in day centres and care homes (see Moniz-Cook 2006 for an overview). Further research should examine exactly which cognitive and psychological features of Cognitive Stimulation intervention are particularly effective, and what (sub)groups of patients benefit most from it. For instance, it is still not known whether the benefits derive mainly from the cognition-focused components, or the social interaction that is a key part of the intervention (Clare and Woods 2004). We outlined in this chapter how CS may contribute to the detection of a developing dementia and early support of people who meet the criteria of MCI, irrespective of whether they are at risk of dementia or not.

CS in MCI can, by virtue of its goals, methods and framework, contribute to our ability to differentiate between those who are 'stable' or 'at risk' of developing dementia, through careful observation by a psychologist of within-session performance. This, combined with detailed neuro-psychological testing repeated over time, has the potential for the detection of early Alzheimer's disease.

As a preventative treatment for dementia, CS as an intervention constitutes learning specific cognitive strategies that may delay the onset of dementia through maximising cognitive reserve capacity, or defer the onset of symptoms since it also takes into account the person, the family and the social environment. Therefore CS in MCI may have a dual role in the prevention of dementia. First, it can help prevent extra burden on cognition in MCI, irrespective of whether the person is at risk of developing dementia, and may thus indirectly reduce the risk of further cognitive decline and the onset of dementia. Second, if CS can be used to enhance efficacy in MCI as well as assist people and families to maintain their lifestyle, it may be possible to delay the deteriorative impact on behaviour and daily functioning as dementia develops in those at risk. A review of the evidence for CS and other cognition-orientated, non-pharmacological interventions in MCI is currently under way (Cameron and Clare 2004). A nationwide controlled randomised trial (N = 1000) comparing CS, cognitive rehabilitation, reminiscence and an individual personally tailored intervention 'à la carte' is currently under way in France (Amieva 2006). It aims to evaluate the relative effectiveness of these four psychosocial interventions in mild and moderate Alzheimer's disease, with the primary outcome set at the delay of conversion into moderate-severe and severe dementia. The hypothesis of the investigators is that people with early stage dementia who benefit from one of the four interventions during three months (one and a half hours weekly) will be significantly less at risk of progression to a severe dementia, at 24 months follow-up, compared to those in a control group who did not receive any of the four interventions (Dartigues and Amieva 2006).

References

Albert, M. (2002) 'Preclinical prediction of Alzheimer's disease.' *Neurobiology of Aging 23*, S561.

Amieva, H. (2006) 'National evaluation programme on Cognitive Stimulation, cognitive rehabilitation and reminiscence.' Paper presented at 7th Annual INTERDEM Meeting, Fondation Médéric Alzheimer, 29 June, Paris.

Astell, A. and Bucks, R. (2002) 'Category fluency in AD: generation from common and ad hoc categories.' Paper presented at 8th International Conference on Alzheimer's Disease and Related Disorders (abstract 974), Stockholm.

Bäckman, L. (2002) 'The cognitive transition to Alzheimer's disease.' Paper presented at 8th International Conference on Alzheimer's Disease and Related Disorders (abstract 1052), Stockholm.

Blackwell, A., Sahakian, B. and Versey, R. (2002) 'Early detection of Alzheimer's disease using neuropsychological assessment: paired associates learning and graded naming.' Paper presented at 8th International Conference on Alzheimer's Disease and Related Disorders (abstract 143), Stockholm.

Bozoki, A., Giordiani, B., Heidebrink, J.L., Berent, S. and Foster, N.L. (2001) 'Mild cognitive Impairment predicts dementia in non-demented elderly patients with memory loss.' *Archives of Neurology 58*, 411–416.

Breuil, V., de Rotrou, J., Forette, F., Tortrat, D., Ganansia-Ganem, A. and Frambourt, A. (1994) 'Cognitive Stimulation of patients with dementia. Preliminary results.' *International Journal of Geriatric Psychiatry 9*, 211–217.

Cameron, M.H. and Clare, L. (2004) 'Cognition-based interventions for people with Mild Cognitive impairment (protocol).' *Cochrane Database of Systematic Reviews, Issue 2.* Chichester: Wiley.

Cantegreil-Kallen, I., de Rotrou, J., Gosselin, A., Wenisch, E. and Rigaud, A.S. (2002) 'The role of Cognitive Stimulation in diagnosing Mild-Cognitive-Impairment subjects at risk for Alzheimer-type dementia.' *Brain Aging 2*, 15–19.

Cimétière, C. (1997) *Evaluation d'une prise en charge de la plainte mnésique chez l'adulte âgé.* Mémoire de DESS de Psychologie du développement. Université de Caen. Caen: UFR des Sciences de la vie et du comportement.

Clare, L. and Woods, R.T. (2004) 'Cognitive training and cognitive rehabilitation for people with early-stage Alzheimer's disease: a review.' *Neuropsychological Rehabilitation 14*, 385–401.

Dartigues, J.F. and Amieva, H. (2006) *Essai clinique prospectif comparatif, multicentrique, randomisé, sans insu évaluant quatre thérapies non-médicamenteuses dans la maladie d'Alzheimer.* Protocole d'étude clinique, version n°0.1 20/09/2006. Bordeaux: Centre Hospitalier Universitaire de Bordeaux.

de Rotrou, J. (2001) 'Stimulation et éducation cognitives. Le vieillissement cérébral.' *Gérontologie et Société 97*, 175–192.

de Rotrou, J., Cantegreil-Kallen, I. and Cimétière, C. (2000) 'Evaluation du memo-sénior.' *Rapport pour la Fondation Nationale de Gérontologie (France).*

de Rotrou, J., Cantegreil-Kallen, I., Gosselin, A., Wenisch, E. and Rigaud, A.S. (2002) 'Cognitive Stimulation: a new approach for Alzheimer's disease management.' *Brain Aging 2*, 48–53.

de Rotrou, J., Forette, F., Tortrat, D., Fermanian, J., Hervy, M.P., Boudou, M.R. and Boller, F. (1991) 'Cognitive efficiency profile, description and validation in patients with Alzheimer's disease.' *International Journal of Geriatric Psychiatry 6*, 501–509.

Ferris, S. (2002) 'Monitoring cognition across the spectrum of AD.' Paper presented at 8th International Conference on Alzheimer's Disease and Related Disorders (abstract 1053), Stockholm.

Gosselin, A., de Rotrou, J., Cantegreil-Kallen, I., Wenisch, E., Moulin, C., Bourrellis, C. and Rigaud, A.S. (2003) 'Bénéfices d'une prise en charge globale sure les troubles comportementaux des patients dements institutionalisés.' In *L'Année Gérontologique. Santé et maison de retraite*, Vol. IV. Paris: Editions Serdi.

Moniz-Cook, E. (2006) 'Cognitive Stimulation and dementia.' *Aging and Mental Health 10*, 207–210.

Palmer, K., Bäckman, L., Winblad, B. and Fratiglioni, L. (2002) 'Cognitive impairment, no dementia: is it possible to identify, with high predictivity, subjects at risk of developing dementia in the general population?' Paper presented at 8th International Conference on Alzheimer's Disease and Related Disorders (abstract 1081), Stockholm.

Petersen, R., Smith, G., Waring, S., Ivnik, R., Tangelos, E. and Kokmen, E. (1999) 'Mild cognitive impairment: clinical characterization and outcome.' *Archives of Neurology 56*, 303–308.

Spector, A., Orrell, M., Davies, S. and Woods, B. (1998) 'Reality orientation for dementia: a review of the evidence for its effectiveness.' *The Cochrane Library Database – Systematic Reviews*, Issue 4. Chichester: Wiley.

Verhey, F. and Visser, P. (2000) 'The phenomenology of depression in dementia.' *International Psychogeriatrics 12*, 129–134.

Vidal, J.C., Lavieille-Letan, S., Fleury, A. and de Rotrou, J. (1998) 'Stimulation cognitive et psychosociale des patients déments en institution.' *La revue de Gériatrie 23*, 199–204.

Zanetti, M., Ballabio, C., Abbate, C., Cutaia, C., Vergani, C. and Bergamaschini, L. (2006) 'Mild cognitive impairment subtypes and vascular dementia in community-dwelling elderly people: a 3-year follow-up study.' *Journal of the American Geriatrics Society 54*, 580–586.

Further reading and related references

de Rotrou, J., Wenisch, E., Chausson, C., Dray, F., Faucounau, V. and Rigaud, A.S. (2005) 'Accidental MCI in healthy subjects: a prospective longitudinal study.' *European Journal of Neurology 12*, 879–885.

Farinamd, E., Mantovani, F., Fioravanti, R., Pignatti, R., *et al.* (2006) 'Evaluating two group programmes of cognitive training in mild to moderate AD: Is there any difference between "global" stimulation and a cognitive-specific one?' *Aging and Mental Health 10*, 211–218.

Knapp, M., Thorgrimsen, L., Patel, A., Spector, A., *et al.* (2006) 'Cognitive Stimulation therapy for people with dementia: cost effectiveness analysis.' *British Journal of Psychiatry 188*, 574–580.

Spector, A., Davies, S., Woods, R.T. and Orrell, M. (2002) 'Reality orientation for dementia: a systematic review of the evidence for its effectiveness.' *Gerontologist 40*, 206–212.

Spector, A., Orrell, M., Davies, S. and Woods, R.T. (2001) 'Can reality orientation be rehabilitated? Development and piloting of an evidence-based programme of cognition-based therapies for people with dementia.' *Neuropsychological Rehabilitation 11*, 377–397.

Spector, A., Thorgrimsen, L., Woods, R.T., Royan, L., *et al.* (2003) 'Efficacy of an evidence-based Cognitive Stimulation therapy programme for people with dementia: randomised controlled trial.' *British Journal of Psychiatry 183*, 248–254.

Spector, A., Thorgrimsen, L., Woods, R.T. and Orrell, M. (2006) *Making a Difference: An Evidence Based Group Programme to Offer Cognitive Stimulation Therapy (CST) to People with Dementia. A Manual for Group Leaders.* London: Hawker Publications.

Woods, B., Thorgrimsen, L., Spector, A., Royan, L. and Orrell, M. (2006) 'Improved quality of life and Cognitive Stimulation therapy in dementia.' *Aging and Mental Health 10*, 219–226.

Chapter 6

GRADIOR

A Personalised Computer-based Cognitive Training Programme for Early Intervention in Dementia

Manuel Franco, Kate Jones,
Bob Woods and Pablo Gomez

Overview

The use of computer technology for rehabilitation in dementia is developing, with a recent pilot randomised study from Spain indicating that multimedia based cognitive stimulation shows promise (Tárraga *et al.* 2006). One such example of computer technology has been developed by a team in northern Spain and used in Wales. This used a specialised computerised programme to assist in cognitive rehabilitation. The programme generated personalised exercises for cognitive training using a compensation perspective to focus on neuropsychological functions and preserved abilities. This has promise as a new tool in early intervention and shows flexibility for use in both urban and rural settings. This chapter outlines a rationale for computer-based neuropsychological rehabilitation programmes in early dementia and the development of this particular system called GRADIOR, in Spain. The application of GRADIOR as part of dementia treatment in Spain and Wales is described using two case studies.

Background

Cognitive rehabilitation for people with dementia uses strategies to either compensate for, or to restore, lost function, particularly in respect of memory deficits. Compensation strategies often use external or environmental aids such as diaries and alarm clocks. Strategies for the restoration of lost function use techniques designed to stimulate deficient mnemonic abilities through repetitive practice, based on the idea that practice can improve the retention of information. The rationale underpinning repetitive practice techniques originated from the idea that the brain can be likened to a mental muscle, and that repetitive mental exercise can strengthen and restore functional deficits. However, effects for people with early dementia tend to be limited and specific to the material that is being processed, with little evidence that improvements generalise to everyday functioning. Thus, whilst repetitive practice using meaningless stimuli is of limited benefit in memory rehabilitation, repetition or rehearsal techniques have been used to good effect for certain types of information. For example, the spaced retrieval technique developed by Landauer and Bjork (1978) involves repeated rehearsal of the 'to be learned information' over increasing delay periods. This technique has been used successfully with people with Alzheimer's disease who learned names and the location of objects and retained this knowledge for several weeks (see, for example, Camp 1989; Camp and McKitrick 1992).

The advent of the computer age has brought a growing interest in the applicability and efficacy of computer-based rehabilitation training including, in recent years, application in the rehabilitation of older people with organic brain disease (Matthews, Harley and Malec 1991). A number of computer systems have been developed for such rehabilitation. Panza *et al.* (1996) used a computer programme that included exercises specifically designed to train and test different facets of memory such as prospective, working, verbal and visuospatial memory using a touch screen monitor. Significant improvement on memory test scores (immediate and delayed memory) were found for people with dementia at the end of the 12-week intervention period. Hofmann, Hock and Müller-Spahn (1996) also found positive effects of an interactive computer-based programme that trained people with mild to moderate Alzheimer's disease. Using photographs of the person with dementia and his or her personal surroundings, an everyday task of relevance to the person was simulated on a PC touch screen, which the patient was trained to operate. After three weeks of training (three to four sessions a week), people needed less help in performing the programmes, they became faster, and the majority made fewer mistakes. Although the training was generally well received, there was no evidence of a general cognitive improvement, and it was uncertain as to whether the results could be transferred to real-life situations.

Positive effects of computer-based rehabilitation were also reported by Schreiber *et al.* (1999) for people with mild to moderate dementia undergoing a training programme designed to improve immediate and delayed retention of objects and routes. The computer tasks simulated real life situations, for example, finding objects in a room, route finding in a virtual house and performing everyday actions such as making a cup of coffee. Training comprised ten 30-minute computer-based sessions with a therapist present to assist where necessary. Members of the control group met with a psychologist in order to control for social stimulation across the two groups and all participants were assessed pre and post test using a variety of neuropsychological tests. The experimental group showed significant improvements on measures of retention of meaningful material and topographical information compared to the control group. However, there were no improvements in retention of meaningless information. This suggested that improvements were domain specific as targeted by the retraining programme. In addition, generalisation to real-life settings was reported for some people, who were verbally provided with a route and were then able to go for a walk and remember the route. The authors argued that cognitive retraining programmes with high ecological validity may facilitate the transfer of cognitive improvements from training to real-life situations.

The effects of cognitive retraining have been found to generalise to broad areas of memory and thinking (Butti *et al.* 1998). Using a multimedia format presenting visual and auditory stimuli that focused on the development of a training package specific to a particular individual, 12 people with vascular dementia participated in five hours cognitive training per week, for ten weeks. Following a period of nine months without training, people once again attended 50 hours of training spaced over ten weeks. Neuropsychological testing was carried out before and after the two training episodes. The programme itself consisted of general attention and memory tasks. Memory and attention exercises were delivered at several levels of difficulty. Once the existing performance levels were established, people were encouraged to attempt the next level of difficulty, thus attempting to train individuals to the limit of their cognitive ability (Butti *et al.* 1998). There were significant improvements in logical memory, visual reproduction and paired associate learning, although this was not maintained at follow-up. A recent pilot randomised clinical trial involving 46 people with Alzheimer's disease from Barcelona, Spain (Tárraga *et al.* 2006) used an Interactive Multimedia Cognitive Stimulation (IMCS) programme called Smartbrain. Participants in the study attended a psychomotor stimulation day care centre and were taking a cholinesterase inhibitor (ChEI). They received a total of 72 multimedia sessions, three times a week lasting a maximum of 25 minutes, over 24 weeks. IMCS was compared with an equivalent group who received Cognitive Psychomotor Stimulation (CPS) at the day care setting and a group that received ChEI alone. At 24-week follow-up the groups who received cognitive stimulation performed better than the ChEI only group on measures of cognition and the group who received additional multimedia cognitive training showed superior outcomes for cognition.

Although memory training may have potential in early dementia support (Bäckman 1992), especially if tailored to the needs and environment of the individual, difficulties exist when introducing such programmes in clinical settings. First, programmes can be seen as costly on therapist time and therefore too expensive to justify. Second, applying a programme can require specific skills and specialised training, as not all psychologists, physicians or occupational therapists may have the knowledge or experience needed. Third, in Spain at least, there are few qualified specialists, so developing a specialised neuropsychological rehabilitation service is difficult. Fourth, there are few theoretically based cognitive training programmes. Fifth, comparison of the best method of maintaining gains at follow-up is not easy to establish. Sixth, when people live some distance from the service, for example, in a rural area, it can be difficult to follow them up and maintain the programme. Finally, the progressive nature of cognitive impairment in people with dementia can impact on professionals who may become overwhelmed by the numbers of people affected. The increasing numbers of older people with dementia that are detected can result in demands for more time for neuropsychological assessment and reporting results, which may ultimately lead to burnout among practitioners (Brooks *et al.* 1999). Box 6.1 outlines what may be needed by developing neuropsychological rehabilitation programmes in dementia to overcome these obstacles.

Box 6.1 Overcoming practical obstacles to the application of neuropsychological rehabilitation programmes in dementia

A programme should be:	
Flexible	Useful for people at many different levels of cognitive impairment.
Open	The programme must be able to easily incorporate any new advances in neuropsychological rehabilitation.
Simple	The programme will need to be applied by those without special qualifications in this area, such as nurses and care workers, so that the neuropsychologist is required only to set up the therapy programme and evaluate its effects.
Available	The programme needs to be accessible and made available for both urban and rural community care services.
Affordable	The programme needs to be inexpensive if its use is to be encouraged.
Useful	The programme must have meaning for the person with dementia and carer and be effective.

Computer-based programmes can meet most of these characteristics and have the following advantages in cognitive stimulation (Seron and Lories 1996):

- Cognitive exercises can be set up and switched on automatically, with varied trials generated by the computer, thus reducing boredom for staff and users.

- Computers are able to give feedback immediately after the user's response, which can enhance motivation.

- Because the user can continue the training at home, more extensive training becomes possible. A computer is needed which can be managed online, so that even those who live far from the specialist rehabilitation centre can participate.

However, computers do have their problems (Matthews et al. 1991; Olbrich 1996; Robertson 1990), not least compatibility issues between different types of software and hardware. In addition, many computer-based rehabilitation programmes are often too rigid to allow modification of cognitive exercises, or there are constraints due to what the programme has been specifically designed to do. Therefore it can be difficult to adapt the memory training to an individual's specific cognitive impairment, without involving a computer specialist. Furthermore, the programmes themselves can be expensive to buy, thus maintaining the perceived high cost of neuropsychological rehabilitation.

The development of GRADIOR

GRADIOR[1] was developed by the INTRAS Foundation in Spain to overcome some of the obstacles to cognitive training in dementia outlined above. GRADIOR is a multimedia system specifically designed for cognitive assessment and neuropsychological rehabilitation which requires only a standard multimedia computer and touch screen (Franco et al. 2000). The user does not therefore need knowledge of how to operate a computer since responses are made via the touch screen. The system can be used in both urban and rural areas, and has been developed to enhance flexibility, new knowledge, use by any practitioner, affordability and utility. It is based on the principle of compensation, i.e. focusing on neuropsychological functions that are still preserved or on those that have least deteriorated. In this way, rehabilitation does not focus exclusively on deficiencies or loss, but more on the abilities which the person has already developed. The programme can be graded and totally personalised, taking into account both environmental and emotional factors.

The GRADIOR system includes three modules as follows:

1. *The exercise generator.*

   o The therapist can build specific, individualised exercises for cognitive training.

2. *The clinic manager programme.*

   o The therapist collects general clinical information on the person with dementia: socio-demographic details, treatments and scores on assessment measures (for example, the Mini Mental State Exam, MMSE; Barthel Index).

   o In designing the treatment, the therapist chooses the specific cognitive exercises for the individual and the number required, and establishes the level of difficulty of every exercise. In this way, the therapist can therefore personalise the memory training to each person's strengths and needs.

   o Verbal and auditory feedback (negative, positive and neutral) are automatically provided throughout each trial and the data are automatically stored for each person, allowing later access to information about each session, together with responses to individual trials. This report facility allows the therapist to evaluate the rehabilitation programme.

3. *The cognitive training application.*

   o The person with dementia works with the computer and carries out different exercises as part of the rehabilitation session.

   o Using a standard set of exercises, it is also possible to carry out a neuropsychological assessment or reassessment.

The system contains a wide variety of exercises designed to tap into distinct cognitive domains including memory, attention, perception and language. Within each cognitive domain the exercises are graded in level of difficulty by manipulation of the number of stimuli, presentation time and inter-stimulus interval. The system separates the content of the exercises from the cognitive activities to be practised. It has a wide selection of pictures, images, sounds and phrases which can be included in different exercises. Each cognitive activity or function is related to an exercise (i.e. practice) module and there is provision for the therapist to build in individually tailored exercises by linking the specific content (for example, the picture, sounds and instructions) with the exercise module. The system then generates the exercises (see Box 6.2). Exercises of varying difficulties can be incorporated into a session that can be tailored to the individual, and stimuli can be added that are personally relevant (for example, familiar faces, events or places).

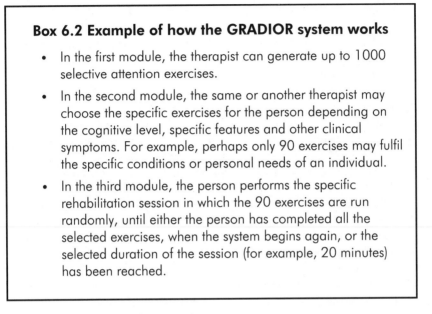

Box 6.2 Example of how the GRADIOR system works

- In the first module, the therapist can generate up to 1000 selective attention exercises.

- In the second module, the same or another therapist may choose the specific exercises for the person depending on the cognitive level, specific features and other clinical symptoms. For example, perhaps only 90 exercises may fulfil the specific conditions or personal needs of an individual.

- In the third module, the person performs the specific rehabilitation session in which the 90 exercises are run randomly, until either the person has completed all the selected exercises, when the system begins again, or the selected duration of the session (for example, 20 minutes) has been reached.

Application of GRADIOR

Originally developed and used in Spain at the INTRAS Foundation, the programme has also been adapted for use in the UK at the University of Wales, Bangor. In Spain it has been used to improve the quality of neuropsychological assessment that in turn can target particular cognitive strengths and needs of the person with dementia in cognitive rehabilitation. In Wales it has also been used for developing cognitive stimulation training activity programmes. Computer-based rehabilitation and outcomes using GRADIOR in two studies from Spain and Wales are described in the following sections of this chapter.

Case example – Adam (Spain)

Adam, aged 77, arrived at the service seeking help with memory and concentration difficulties. He felt these hindered some of his everyday activities and he described his poor performance at his weekend job, which required him to receive telephone calls and take currency-changing orders solicited by various city firms. He observed that the order forms would become increasingly full of ink blots and he needed to repeat the operation many times to take the 'message' correctly. He also reported symptoms of slight dizziness at specific moments, for example, when going up the stairs, and that relatives had begun to note slight absentmindedness which, without interfering too much in everyday life, was nonetheless significant. At the first session, subclinical depressive symptoms of one year duration were noted, probably associated with Adam's subjective feeling of being incapable due to initial forgetfulness, and later with a more notable functional memory loss.

An exhaustive analysis of his presenting symptoms was undertaken based on organic neuropsychological protocols. Medical explorations included routine blood and urine tests, electroencephalography (EEG) and computerised tomography (CT) scan, all of which were normal. Neuropsychological exploration also provided a baseline assessment prior to cognitive rehabilitation. A number of cognitive tests were used in this initial evaluation including the: Mini Cognitive Examination (Lobo et al., 1979, 1980), Alzheimer's Disease Assessment Scale (ADAS) test (Rosen, Mohs and Davis 1984) and the Clock Drawing Test (Freeman et al. 1994). Additionally, a series of tests aimed at assessing mood, self-esteem, functional ability, quality of life for the patient, depression and quality of life among the person's relatives were used included the Lawton Scale (Lawton and Brody 1972), Barthel Index (Mahoney and Barthel 1965) and the Clinician's Global Impressions (see Schneider and Olin 1997).

The initial evaluation found evidence of mild cognitive deterioration, mild dementia of Alzheimer type, and difficulties with independent daily living. Alzheimer's disease with no associated behavioural or mood disorder was diagnosed. Adam did not wish to take an anti-dementia drug, but used GRADIOR for a year. Box 6.3 outlines the effects of rehabilitation with GRADIOR for Adam and his wife.

Case example – Paula (Wales)

Paula is a 72-year-old woman who was admitted to a specialist assessment unit with memory problems that had impacted on her daily living. She was aware of having some memory difficulties. Neuropsychological assessment indicated the following: her performance on the Cambridge Cognitive Examination for Mental Disorders – Revised (CAMCOG-R) (Roth et al. 1988) was 32/105 (the mean for someone of this age is 88.3); MMSE (Folstein, Folstein and McHugh 1975) score was 7/30 and she was greatly impaired on orientation and recent memory. On tests of frontal lobe functioning Paula performed poorly on abstract thinking and visual reasoning. Overall, the cognitive assessment suggested that Paula had a severe impairment, with her comprehension and expression abilities being less impaired than her other cognitive skills. Box 6.4 describes Paula's use of the GRADIOR computerised rehabilitation programme.

Figure 6.1 shows that, despite Paula's significantly reduced level of cognitive impairment, she was able to learn how to respond appropriately to the trials and showed consistent improvement over the seven sessions.

Box 6.3 Adam and his wife: rehabilitation with GRADIOR

Adam participated in 25-minute GRADIOR sessions held twice weekly for a year. The programme was personalised to domains of attention, memory and information processing. Assessments were made at 3, 6, 9 and 12 months after commencing rehabilitation and some of the outcome results are shown below.

RESULTS	Mini cognitive exam	ADAS test			Clock drawing test	Lawton	Barthel	Clinicians' global impression	
		Non-cog.	Cog.	Total				Evaluator	Family
Baseline	24	14	9	23	16	5	95	2	2
3 months	34				17			2	2
6 months	29	16	2	18	16	5	95	2	2
9 months	33				18			2	2
12 months	33	12	4	16	18	5	95	2	2

- There were improvements in cognitive functioning reflecting target domains.

- There were associated positive effects on everyday life, particularly performance in carrying out his job (taking orders by phone). Qualitative examination of the order forms indicated that these no longer had as many ink blots or scribbles and he reported that he did not have to repeat the order as many times to get it right.

- His mood also improved (ADAS non-cog), probably due to improved self-esteem (measures for mood and self-esteem are available from first author). This appeared to have been reinforced by his experiences of success in his cognitive training programme and more importantly in his everyday life, particularly his weekend job – he was pleased with his achievements.

- There were additional positive effects on his wife's reported burden and the quality of her life did not worsen over the 12 months (measures are available from first author).

Box 6.4 Paula – intervention with GRADIOR

Paula participated in seven 20-minute GRADIOR sessions held twice weekly over a four-week period. The GRADIOR programme was presented on a PC and Microtouch software was used to activate the touch screen. The sessions took place in a quiet office. Initially, Paula was presented with a session comprising a mixture of level one exercises targeting perception, memory and attention skills. During the first session additional verbal instructions were given wherever necessary. In subsequent sessions minimal instructions were given.

Conclusion

Interactive multimedia tools for cognitive stimulation in dementia are developing, such as the programme Smartbrain (www.educamigos.com, accessed 7 August 2008), which has 19 stimulation tasks at different levels of difficulty across the range of cognitive domains. This has been piloted in a recent randomised trial of cognitive stimulation (Tárraga et al. 2006). We have described another such tool, GRADIOR, which extends generalised cognitive stimulation to a more targeted personalised cognitive rehabilitative programme. GRADIOR has the potential to improve the quality of neuropsychological assessment and assist with personalised cognitive training, including ongoing evaluation, on particular domains of cognition. Training in dementia rehabilitation can be wide ranging and geared to the person's expressed wishes. It may focus on broader cognitive stimulation as a means of activity programmes for people in early stage dementia who are aware of their problems and wish to do something about them. It may also be useful as a domain-specific targeted cognitive rehabilitation programme by developing restorative strategies for a particular domain or to improve everyday performance, such as rehearsing where important items are stored or an important route. GRADIOR has been used for dementia rehabilitation in urban and rural settings and in specialised assessment centres (Wales, UK) and non-specialised settings such as a health centre or the person's home (Spain). The extent of the stimuli available allows for graded programming that can maintain a person's motivation, encourage regular use of the memory training system, and maintain memory efficacy and competence. Involving family carers in memory stimulation with GRADIOR in the home can also assist them in combating their widely reported concerns of apathy in their relative with early dementia. In this chapter we have described its use in compensatory strategies. GRADIOR also offers a flexible, interactive and supportive programme between the person with dementia and the computer and it can, if this is what a patient or family wishes, be used for domain-specific restoration. A recent meta-analysis of cognitive training in

Percentage of correct responses over 7 sessions

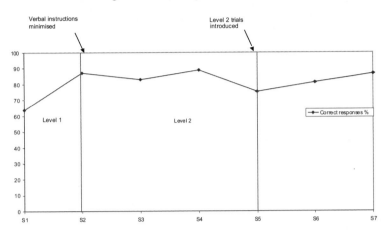

Figure 6.1 Effect of GRADIOR on Paula

Errors: A fine grained analysis of the errors by type of exercise revealed that Paula did not produce errors in the perception exercises. A paired t test revealed a significantly higher error rate for attention trials (M = 10.85) than for memory trials (M = 4.57), t (5) = 2.88, p<0.02.

Attention performance: most of the errors were present in attention exercises. Persistent problems were noted for exercises that involved auditory selection of a letter embedded in a spoken letter sequence, vigilance tasks and stimulus detection. Visual selective attention tasks consistently proved less problematic as they showed the lowest error rate across all the sessions.

One explanation for why Paula found the auditory task problematic is that these exercises also involve a memory component. For example, a target letter is heard and displayed briefly on the screen. The task is then to attend to a list of spoken letters and to respond when the target letter is heard again. This obviously involves working memory, and people who have memory deficits as well as attention problems may well find this task exceptionally difficult.

Memory performance: More problems were apparent for tasks that involved delayed recognition memory (i.e. the compound delayed recognition task proved more difficult). This was in contrast to simple delayed tasks, where the target words or pictures appear on the screen in a grid intermixed with non-target words and the compound task involves presentation of a sequence of target and non-target words requiring a yes or no response to be made to each individual word or picture. For example, at level one two words were presented and Paula had few problems in recalling immediate and simple delayed recognition tasks whilst errors were consistently made in the compound delayed tasks. This pattern was similar when level two tasks that involved recognition of three target words or pictures were introduced.

Comment: The pattern indicates that although Paula appears to have little difficulty in perception of stimuli, she had marked difficulties in delayed recall and attention. Although cognitive assessment suggested that she had severe impairments, Paula was able to comprehend instructions, engage and interact with the programme. Despite a short intervention period, Paula showed an improvement over time for level one and level two exercises, suggesting that people presenting with memory problems in a clinical setting can improve in task-specific cognitive processing (Franco *et al.* 1998). Paula appeared to enjoy doing the exercises and no particular problems with its implementation were noted.

Alzheimer's disease suggests that, compared with compensatory strategies, restorative programmes have a greater effect on overall functioning (Sitzer, Twamley and Jeste 2006).

Note

1   Available from first author by email at intras@intras.es.

Acknowledgements

Teresa Orihuela and Yolanda Bueno for assistance in developing and evaluating GRADIOR at INTRAS in Spain.

References

Bäckman, L. (1992) 'Memory training and memory improvement in Alzheimer's disease: rules and exceptions.' *Acta Neurologica Scandinavica 139*, 84–89.

Brooks, J.O., Friedman, L., Pearman, A.M., Gray, C. and Yesavage, J.A. (1999) 'Mnemonic training in older adults: effects of age, length of training and type of cognitive pre-training.' *International Psychogeriatrics 11*, 75–84.

Butti, G., Buzzelli, S., Fiori, M. and Giaquito, S. (1998) 'Observations on mentally impaired elderly patients treated with THINKable, a computerised cognitive remediation.' *Archives of Gerontology and Geriatrics 6*, 49–56.

Camp, C.J. (1989) 'Facilitation of New Learning in Alzheimer's Disease.' In G.C. Gilmore, P.J. Whitehouse and M.L. Wykle (eds) *Memory, Aging, and Dementia: Theory, Assessment, and Treatment.* New York, NY: Springer.

Camp, C.J. and McKitrick, L.A. (1992) 'Memory Interventions in DAT Populations: Methodological and Theoretical Issues.' In R.L. West and J.L. Sinnott (eds) *Everyday Memory and Aging: Current Research and Methodology.* New York, NY: Springer-Verlag.

Folstein, M., Folstein, S. and McHugh, P.R. (1975) 'Mini-Mental State Exam (MMSE): a practical method for grading the cognitive state of patients for the clinician.' *Journal of Psychiatric Research 12*, 189–198.

Franco, M., Orihuela, T., Bueno, Y., Gomez, P., Gonzalez, D. and Woods, B. (2000) 'Computers for memory training.' *Journal of Dementia Care 8*, 14.

Freeman, M., Leach, L., Kaplan, E., Winocur, G., Shulman, K.L. and Delis, D.C. (1994) *Clock Drawing: A Neuropsychological Analysis.* Oxford: Oxford University Press.

Hofmann, M., Hock, C. and Müller-Spahn, F. (1996) 'Interactive computer-based cognitive training in patients with Alzheimer's disease.' *Journal of Psychiatric Research 30*, 493–501.

Landauer, T.K. and Bjork, R.A. (1978) 'Optimum Rehearsal Patterns and Name Learning.' In M.M. Gruneberg, P.E. Morris and R.N. Sykes (eds) *Practical Aspects of Memory.* London: Academic Press.

Lawton, M.P. and Brody, E.M. (1972) 'Assessment of Older People.' In D. Kent, R. Kastenbaum and S. Sherwood (eds) *Research, Planning and Action for the Elderly.* New York, NY: Behavioral Publications.

Lobo, A., Ezquerra, J., Gomez-Burgada, F., Sala, J.M. and Seva, A. (1979) 'El Mini-Examen Cognoscitivo (un test sencillo, práctico, para detectar alteraciones intelectuales en pacientes médicos).' *Actas luso-españolas de Neurología, Psiquiatría y Ciencias afines 3*, 189–202.

Lobo, A., Escolar, V., Esquerra, J. and Seva, A. (1980) 'Mini-Examen Cognoscitivo: un test sencillo y práctico para detectar alteraciones intelectivas en pacientes psiquiátricos.' *Revista Psiquiatría y Psicología Medica 5*, 39–57.

Mahoney, F.I. and Barthel, D.W. (1965) 'Functional evaluation: the Barthel Index.' *Maryland State Medical Journal 14*, 61–65.

Matthews, C.G., Harley, J.P.Y. and Malec, J.F. (1991) 'Guidelines for computer-assisted neuropsychological rehabilitation and cognitive remediation.' *The Clinical Neuropsychologist 5*, 3–19.

Olbrich, R. (1996) 'Computer based psychiatric rehabilitation: current activities in Germany.' *European Psychiatry 11*, 60–65.

Panza, V., Solfrizzi, F., Mastroianni, G.A., Cigliola, F. and Capruso, A. (1996) 'A rehabilitation program for mild memory impairments.' *Archives of Gerontology and Geriatrics 5*, 51–55.

Robertson, I. (1990) 'Does computerized cognitive rehabilitation work? A review.' *Aphasiology 4*, 381–405.

Rosen, W.G., Mohs, R.C. and Davis, K.L. (1984) 'A new rating scale for Alzheimer's disease.' *American Journal of Psychiatry 141*, 1356–1364.

Roth, M., Huppert, F.A., Mountjoy, C.Q. and Tym, E. (1988) *CAMDEX-R: The Cambridge Examination for Mental Disorders of the Elderly – Revised.* Cambridge: Cambridge University Press.

Schneider, L.S. and Olin, J.T. (1997) 'Clinical global impressions in Alzheimer's clinical trials.' *International Psychogeriatrics 8*, 277–288.

Schreiber, M., Schweizer, A., Lutz, K., Kalveram, K.T. and Jaencke, L. (1999) 'Potential of an interactive computer-based training in the rehabilitation of dementia: an initial study.' *Neuropsychological Rehabilitation 9*, 155–167.

Seron, X. and Lories, G. (1996) 'El apoyo de la computadora en al valoración y rehabilitación neuropsocológica.' In O. Ostrosky-Solis, A. Ardila and R. Chayo-Dichy (eds) *Rehabilitación Neuropsicológica.* Méjico: Planeta.

Sitzer, D.I., Twamley, E.W. and Jeste, D.V. (2006) 'Cognitive training in Alzheimer's disease: a meta-analysis of the literature.' *Acta Psychiatrica Scandinavica 114*, 75–90.

Tárraga, L., Boada, M., Modinos, G., Espinosa, A., *et al.* (2006) 'A randomised pilot study to assess the efficacy of an interactive, multimedia tool of cognitive stimulation in Alzheimer's disease.' *Journal of Neurology, Neurosurgery and Psychiatry 77*, 1116–1121.

Further reading and related references

Alm, N., Astell, A., Ellis, M., Dye, R., Gowans, G. and Campbell, J. (2004) 'A Cognitive Prosthesis and Communication Support for People with Dementia.' In P. Gregor and A. Newell (eds) *Neuropsychological Rehabilitation: Technology in Cognitive Rehabilitation.* Hove: Psychology Press.

Clare, L. and Woods, R.T. (2001) *Cognitive Rehabilitation in Dementia.* Hove: Psychology Press.

Clare, L. and Woods, R.T. (2004) 'Cognitive training and cognitive rehabilitation for people with early Alzheimer's disease. A review.' *Neuropsychological Rehabilitation 14*, 385–401.

Clare, L., Woods, B., Moniz-Cook, E., Orrell, M. and Spector, A. (2003) 'Cognitive rehabilitation and cognitive training interventions targeting memory functioning in early stage Alzheimer's disease and vascular dementia (review)'. In *The Cochrane Database of Systematic Reviews*, Issue 4. Chichester: Wiley.

Franco, M.A. and Orihuela, T. (1998) *Programa AIRE. Sistema Multimedia de Evaluación y Entrenamiento Cerebral.* Valladolid: Edintras.

Franco, M.A., Orihuela, T., Bueno, Y. and Cid, T. (2000) *Programa Gradior: Programa de Evaluación y Rehabilitación cognitiva por ordenador.* Valladolid: Edintras.

Glisky, E.L. (1995) 'Computers in Memory Rehabilitation.' In A.D. Baddeley, B.A. Wilson and Watts, F.N. (eds) *Handbook of Memory Disorders.* Chichester: Wiley.

Gregor, P. and Newell, A. (eds) (2004) 'Technology in cognitive rehabilitation.' *Neuropsychological Rehabilitation 14*, 1–2, 1–256.

Kapur, N., Glisky, E.L. and Wilson, B.A. (2004a) 'External Memory Aids and Computers in Memory Rehabilitation.' In A.D. Baddeley, M. Kopelman and B.A. Wilson (eds) *The Essential Memory Handbook of Memory Disorders for Clinicians.* Chichester: Wiley.

Kapur, N., Glisky, E.L. and Wilson, B.A. (2004b) 'Technological memory aids for people with memory deficits.' *Neuropsychological Rehabilitation 14*, 1–2, 41–60.

Quittre, A., Olivier C. and Salmon, E. (2005) 'Compensating strategies for impaired episodic memory and time orientation in a patient with Alzheimer's disease.' *Acta Neurologica Belgica 105*, 30–38.

Smartbrain. www.educamigos.com/educamigos/sta/index.jsp (accessed 7 August 2008).

Chapter 7

Memory Groups for People with Early Dementia

Molly Burnham

Overview

Memory problems in dementia can affect an individual's day-to-day life in many ways. For example, daily routines and activities such as shopping, managing money, using public transport, cooking or finding one's way around can become difficult for the individual. Meeting new people and socialising can at times be awkward, particularly if the person with the memory impairment cannot remember recent conversations or people they have been introduced to. Such memory 'failures' in daily life can have an impact on self-confidence and well-being. Therefore it is important that people with memory problems are supported, in order that they can maintain a satisfying and meaningful lifestyle. Memory group therapy is one way to support people in early stage dementia with their memory difficulties. This chapter will describe a memory group therapy course and its effectiveness in helping people continue to live as near normal lives as possible. It will also discuss methods of assessment that are necessary in determining an individual's suitability for a memory group based course.

Memory impairment is typically the earliest manifestation of most dementias. The question of learning how to cope with and respond to these memory difficulties is very likely to arise for the majority of those afflicted. Carers are also just as likely to express strong emotions about the memory problems, such as frustration, anger, fear or sadness and may also need advice on how to cope with memory problems (Clare 1999). It is important that some form of psychosocial intervention is implemented so as to optimise functioning and well-being of the person with dementia, minimise the risk of excess disability, and to prevent the development of a 'malignant social psychology' (Kitwood 1997). Cognitive training and cognitive rehabilitation are the main interventions used with people who are in the early stages of dementia (Clare and Woods 2004). Indeed, McEvoy and Patterson (1986) assessed the effectiveness of a short-term training programme designed to return institutionalised people with Alzheimer's disease back into the community, and participants showed improvement in most areas of personal information, spatial orientation, communication and activities of daily living. However, more complex activities such as money management or meal selection did not improve with training. Furthermore, Piccolini *et al.* (1992) demonstrated improvements in cognitive functioning with a month-long cognitive training programme for older hospital patients who showed cognitive impairment. However, a more specific memory intervention may take place in a group therapy environment and is a way of supporting people with memory difficulties.

The aim of memory group therapy

The most obvious goal of memory group sessions is to help people with memory problems to overcome their difficulties, by teaching them various strategies and techniques, so that they are able to continue their daily activities as before. Other goals of group therapy are to build confidence, improve socialisation, and promote problem solving. The course aims to introduce people relatively early in their illness to the concept of using memory aids and techniques, so that they can make a habit of using them. Members of the group learn to apply basic principles and techniques of learning and recall in a variety of practical situations, such as getting to know new people. The idea is that once individuals have successfully learnt these principles they will be able to transfer them to other situations. The benefits of a group therapy setting (as opposed to individual therapy) are key to providing the support that people with early dementia need. Such advantages of memory group therapy are as follows:

1. People realise that they are 'not alone' in having memory problems.

2. They are able to accept their personal situation.

3. They encourage each other, offering mutual support, and are able to share successes and failures without embarrassment.

4. Acknowledgement from other members of the group of an individual's progress increases self-esteem.

5. The social aspect of the group is important since people with early dementia often tend to become isolated.

6. The group setting provides time and space in an unthreatening environment within which to practise the skills and techniques learned.

Memory group therapy course

The *basic principles* taught include helping people to learn how to use different memory aids (e.g. calendars, timers, dictaphones and visual prompts) and to decide which will be the most useful for them. The importance of routines and habits is highlighted, and members of the group are encouraged to identify skills which they particularly wish to retain, for example, dressing themselves or playing bowls. The members are then encouraged to 'over-learn' these skills.

The *core techniques* taught and transferred to different areas include repetition, frequent recall, association with something/someone already known, the use of rhymes, alliteration and mnemonics, the use of suitable memory aids, and making use of habits, including the 'over-rehearsal' of important skills. As many senses as possible are involved in the learning process and individuals identify which senses are most useful to them in both the registration and the recall process.

The course is designed as a series of separate topics which are covered in the order most appropriate for the individuals involved (see Box 7.1 for course topics). The handouts are designed specifically for people with memory problems using simple language and pictorial prompts, and participants are encouraged to go over the session handouts with a relative or friend (see Box 7.2 for an example of a handout).

Guidance for introducing a memory group

Although the sessions described here have been developed from an occupational therapy perspective, successful groups can also be run by mental health nurses, psychologists and speech therapists. Between six to ten clients are pre-selected to go to the memory group, and they are encouraged to attend every session. There may be between 6 to 12 sessions, depending on the needs of the group. Ideally, there should be two facilitators to lead interactive groups, to assess the needs of individual members and to monitor their progress. Before and after the group each member should be visited at home to assist in implementing the techniques learnt, helping to improve the person's quality of

Box 7.1 Topics covered on memory group therapy course

CORE SESSIONS

Getting to know you	• Because group members are often people who do not know each other, this activity is normally used at the beginning of the course. • The session looks at the different ways that can be used to learn and recall people's names, and includes a practical name-learning exercise in the group. • Photos may also be taken in order that people can have pictures to help them remember the names of other group members.
How we remember	• Registration, retention and recall are discussed, as well as memory linked to each of the senses. • Group members are encouraged to identify what senses are personally most useful to them. • Different kinds of memory such as semantic, personal and procedural are also introduced, but not named as such.
Hurrah for habits	• This unit covers skills and habits, together with the use of memory aids. • Each person identifies aids that might help them and the group discusses how they can make a habit of using them.
The all-important question	• This topic introduces the use of questions as an aid to concentration at the registration stage, and also as a tool for recall. • A framework of questions to help concentration when listening, reading or planning what to say is introduced, for example, questions starting with who, what, why or when, and suggestions for using it.
Mood and memory	• Often used towards the end of the unit when group members have become very comfortable with each other, this unit discusses the emotional responses to memory impairment and the effect of emotions on registration and recall.

SUPPLEMENTARY UNITS (incorporated according to the different needs of each group)

- Finding your way.
- Telephone talk.
- Money matters.
- Remembering what you read.
- Confidence in the kitchen.
- Sensible shopping.
- Using public transport.

life. Members tend to perform better with carer support, so it is useful if their carers attend carer support groups, since they enable them to become familiar with the material and ways of reinforcing the techniques taught between sessions. However, it must be noted that the presence of carers in the memory group therapy sessions may inhibit group members. Members may also benefit from a monthly follow-up 'memory club' which people who have completed a course may join. These sessions reiterate topics covered on the course and allow members to benefit from individual help both during the sessions and afterwards.

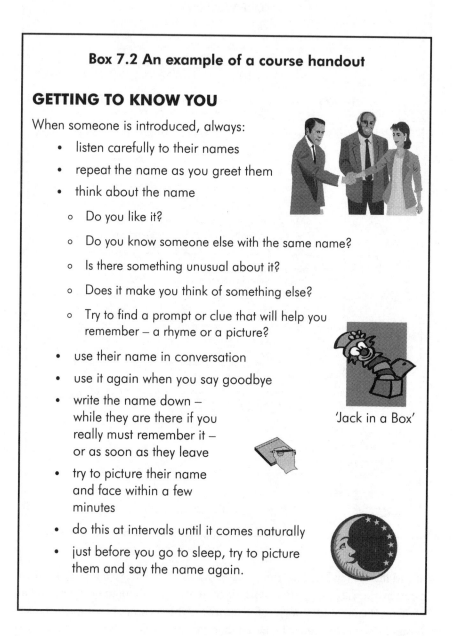

Box 7.2 An example of a course handout

GETTING TO KNOW YOU

When someone is introduced, always:

- listen carefully to their names
- repeat the name as you greet them
- think about the name

  o Do you like it?

  o Do you know someone else with the same name?

  o Is there something unusual about it?

  o Does it make you think of something else?

  o Try to find a prompt or clue that will help you remember – a rhyme or a picture?

- use their name in conversation
- use it again when you say goodbye
- write the name down – while they are there if you really must remember it – or as soon as they leave

'Jack in a Box'

- try to picture their name and face within a few minutes
- do this at intervals until it comes naturally
- just before you go to sleep, try to picture them and say the name again.

Selecting who can benefit from memory groups

It is important that all group members have a similar level of cognitive ability and they recognise that they have a memory problem. They should also have adequate hearing and speech to allow them to participate in the group sessions, and they need to be committed to the group and each other so that they can benefit from the therapy. People are more likely to benefit if they are insightful, motivated, able to communicate within a group setting and are at an early stage in their dementia. Due to the specific inclusion criteria, there has to be careful assessment before the group. There are a number of assessments which can be carried out in order to determine how appropriate it is for an individual to join a memory group.

First, potential members of the memory group should be interviewed to ensure that they recognise they have a memory problem, have no perception difficulties and are keen to participate in such therapy. It is also useful to assess the extent to which the person's carer is supportive of the programme. Second, all potential members should be assessed using, for example, the Mini Mental State Examination (MMSE, Folstein, Folstein and McHugh 1975). Providing the other conditions are met, those who score 22/30 or above will be able to benefit from the memory therapy. Occupational therapists have also found the Large Allen Cognitive Level Screen (LACLS, Allen 1996) and the Assessment of Motor and Process Skills (AMPS) to be more appropriate and sensitive measures. Since formal assessment can be stressful for people, it is recommended that only one of these assessments is used in the screening interview, as well as any other assessment normally used in the care setting. Third, the effectiveness of the intervention may be evaluated using Quality of Life (QOL) assessments and carer questionnaires in order to detect any change. Ideally, assessment should occur before the group starts, soon after completion, three months later and then at six month intervals.

Memory groups for people with early dementia have so far been found to be very effective. The following describes the case of Bernard who was diagnosed with Alzheimer's disease and attended memory group therapy sessions.

Case example – Bernard

Bernard was only 52 when he was diagnosed with Alzheimer's disease. He had gone to his GP because he was no longer coping with a responsible position in an electronics firm. Once he had received his diagnosis, his employer encouraged him to return to work, but in a less demanding position. Bernard was keen to maintain this for as long as possible. He joined a memory group which took place in the evening once a week for seven weeks.

Bernard was tested before and after the group using the Assessment of Motor and Process Skills (AMPS) and the Rivermead Behavioural Memory Test (RBMT, Wilson, Cockburn and Baddeley 1985). Bernard's scores before the group were 2.70 for Motor (physical) Skills (+2 = cut-off point; person can live unaided in the community) and 1.16 for Process (cognitive) Skills (+1 = cut-off point).

After completing the group sessions, these scores had risen to 2.77 and 1.58. The small increase in Motor Skills is probably not significant, but the increase of 0.42 in his Process Skills is a marked improvement. There was an increase of 12 to 15 per cent for Adaptation, Space and Objects, and Using Knowledge (all Process categories). A 10 per cent increase in Strength and Effort outweighed the 9 per cent decrease in his score for Co-ordination (Motor categories).

On the Screening score for the RBMT, Bernard showed an increase of 16.6 per cent, although there was only a small, non-significant, improvement on the Standardised Profile score.

As a result of the group sessions Bernard started using a number of new memory aids and strategies (making lists, using a calendar or diary, reminder notes, shopping list, notebook and prioritising tasks). No doubt these helped him to maintain the performance as shown by retesting a year after the group. When he had new difficulties he discussed these with his wife, and he was able to find a 'trick' to help. He was continuing to meet up with his friends, one of whom would prompt him when it was his turn to buy a round of drinks for his friends at the local pub.

More informal sessions of other groups indicate that when the training takes place early in the course of the illness, and where the core principles have continued to be reinforced, some people have continued to improve even after the formal sessions have ended. Moreover, it appears that those who develop personalised coping strategies during the programme are more likely to maintain their memory skills. For example, one member who was a window cleaner thought he would have to stop work because he went to the same house twice in one week and neglected others. However, he started using a dictaphone to record which windows he cleaned each day and whether he had been paid. This worked very well and he was able to continue in employment. Even when decline continues, once the principles have been learnt they appear to enable more effective functioning for longer. It is therefore evident that memory group therapy does indeed offer a way of support for people with early dementia and allows them to live a more meaningful and satisfying way of life. More research is needed into the long-term effects of memory training and the evaluation of longer lasting courses, but the lack of adverse effects of such group therapy suggests that it has the potential to empower the person to increase their cognitive strengths and to continue finding methods of attaining personally meaningful and important goals (Clare and Woods 2004).

Acknowledgements

The memory therapy course described in this chapter was first piloted in an NHS setting in Buckinghamshire, UK with people below the age of 65 who had been diagnosed with dementia (i.e. 'Young-onset Dementia') between 1995 and 1997. The author would like to acknowledge Denise Cottrell (clinical psychologist) for support with this programme. The work was then re-developed in an NHS setting in Sussex working with older people within an early identification and psychosocial intervention service. The author would like to acknowledge Dr Caroline Williams (clinical psychologist), for supporting this intervention in Sussex.

References

Allen, C.K. (1996) *Allen Cognitive Level Test Manual* (with kit included). Colchester, CT: S&S Worldwide. Available at www.ssww.com, accessed 7 August 2008.

Clare, L. (1999) 'Memory rehabilitation in early dementia.' *Journal of Dementia Care 6*, 33–38.

Clare, L. and Woods, R.T. (2004) 'Cognitive training and cognitive rehabilitation for people with early-stage Alzheimer's disease: a review.' *Neuropsychological Rehabilitation 14*, 385–401.

Folstein, M., Folstein, S. and McHugh, P.R. (1975) 'Mini-Mental State Exam (MMSE): a practical method for grading the cognitive state of patients for the clinician.' *Journal of Psychiatric Research 12*, 189–198.

Kitwood, T. (1997) *Dementia Reconsidered: The Person Comes First.* Maidenhead: Open University Press.

McEvoy, C.L. and Patterson, R.L. (1986) 'Behavioural treatment of deficit skills in dementia patients.' *Gerontologist 26*, 475–478.

Piccolini, C., Amadio, L., Spazzafumo, L., Moroni, S. and Freddi, A. (1992) 'The effects of a rehabilitation program with mnemotechniques on the institutionalised elderly subject.' *Archives of Gerontology and Geriatrics 15*, 141–149.

Wilson, B.A., Cockburn, J. and Baddeley, A.D. (1985) *The Rivermead Behavioural Memory Test.* Bury St Edmunds: Thames Valley Test Company. Available at www.pearson-uk.com, accessed 7 August 2008.

Further reading and related references

Assessment of Motor and Process Skills (AMPS). For further information on this standardised assessment see www.ampsintl.com (accessed 7 August 2008).

Burnham, M. (1999) 'Effective group memory therapy for people with dementia.' *Signpost 3*, 4, 12–14.

Gordon, B. (1995) *Memory: Remembering and Forgetting in Everyday Life.* New York, NY: MasterMedia Ltd.

Nichols, R. and Cole, A. (1999) 'Nurse led – an accessible memory service.' *Signpost 4*, 3, 37–39.

Rupp, R. (1998) *Committed to Memory: How We Remember and Why We Forget.* London: Aurum Press.

Wilson, B.A. and Moffat, N. (1992) 'The Development of Group Memory Therapy.' In B.A. Wilson and N. Moffat (eds) *Clinical Management of Memory Problems*, 2nd edn. San Diego, CA: Singular Publishing Group.

Winter, A. and Winter, R. (1997) *Brain Workout: Easy Ways to Power Up Your Memory, Sensory Perception, and Intelligence.* New York, NY: St. Martin's Griffin.

Available resource

The booklets referred to and a facilitator's handbook are available to print out from a CD: *Memory Management Groups for People with Early Stage Dementia* © Molly L. Burnham. This may be obtained from the author. For further information about running memory training groups and to obtain copies of the course material, please email: molly_burnham@hotmail.com or molly.burnham@ntlworld.com

Chapter 8

Health Technologies for People with Early Dementia
The ENABLE Project

Suzanne Cahill, Emer Begley and Inger Hagen

Overview

ENABLE was a European longitudinal study carried out in five countries, namely Norway, Ireland, the UK, Finland and Lithuania. The study started in March 2000 and was funded by the European Commission under the programme for Quality of Life and Management of Living Resources (File No QLK6–CT-2000–00653). The overall aim of ENABLE was to investigate whether it was possible to facilitate more independent living for people with mild to moderate dementia and promote their quality of life, by installing at-home assistive technologies. This would be done by evaluating both the individual and his or her family carer's experiences of using these products over a 12-month period. The specific aims of ENABLE were as follows:

- to examine whether assistive technologies can enable people with dementia by supporting their well-being, giving positive experiences, reducing worries and unrest, and reducing the burden of carers

- to develop a methodology to assess the effects of providing assistive technologies to people with dementia living at home

- to develop approaches to assessing the socio-economic costs and benefits of developing, implementing and using assistive technologies

- to investigate cross-country differences and similarities in the feasibility of devices and in applying methodologies to their assessment.

This chapter presents findings from the Irish assessment study for ENABLE, six months after product installation first took place. In particular, the chapter reports on outcome variables (dependent) including use and usefulness of these products both from a family carer's perspective and from that of the person diagnosed with dementia. Some case studies are also drawn on to capture, in more depth, the complexities of the lives of people diagnosed with dementia in order to better understand their particular problems coping with dementia and adapting to these new psychosocial interventions.

Background

Dementia carries a heavy economic burden, not only for all those diagnosed with the illness but for their primary carers, the community and society at large. The disability weight for dementia is higher than for almost any other health condition, with the exception of terminal cancer and spinal injury (Ferri *et al.* 2005) and the worldwide costs of dementia are significant (Wimo, Jonsson and Winblad 2006). In advanced economies, many of these financial costs are borne by family members, since most people with dementia continue to live at home attempting to manage daily tasks themselves. Accordingly, whilst most people diagnosed wish to live at home, many family carers emphasise the complexities of the home environment, particularly the disabling impact of contemporary technology (Sweep 1998). As the illness progresses many people with dementia experience failures because their ability to maintain relationships or handle activities of daily living progressively deteriorates. Combined, this can lead to poorer physical functioning, depression and a reduced quality of life. Thus, many of the challenges faced by people with dementia and their family carers are of a very practical nature (Bjørneby, Topo and Holthe 1999; Marshall 2000). This has led to a burgeoning interest in the use of in-home technology to support the care and well-being of people with dementia (see, for example, Holthe, Hagen and Bjørneby 1999; Woolham 2006; Woolham *et al.* 2002; *Teknik och demens* [technology and dementia] projects funded by the Swedish Institute of Assistive Technology and the Nordic Development Centre for Rehabilitation Technology, www.hi.se and www.nuh.fi, both accessed 7 August 2008).

The Irish context

According to one Irish expert, the application of Eurodem prevalence rates to the most recent census of population data for Ireland, suggests that there are currently some 34,097 people with dementia living in Ireland of whom 20,222 are women and 13,875 men (O'Shea 2006). While most of these people live at home (O'Shea and O'Reilly 1999a, 1999b), there is no community care legislation in Ireland, placing an onus on the Health Service Executive to provide services to older people with a dementia that are free of charge and as a right (since January 2005, health and personal social services in Ireland are delivered by the Health Service Executive through a network of local health officers, health centres and clinics). Accordingly, apart from a small numbers of universal services (such as free travel and free access to primary care), most core social services in Ireland are delivered in a discretionary ad hoc manner and on a selective rather than universal basis (Gallagher 2006). In this regard and in the context of the current model in Ireland of a mixed economy of welfare, psychosocial interventions by way of assistive technological services for older people including those with dementia, have not been legislated for. Curiously this sets Ireland apart from other European countries such as the UK, Finland and Norway, where legislation for older people's services, including the supply and maintenance of technologies, has been in place for some time. ENABLE was therefore pivotal in Ireland in attempting to raise professional and public awareness about the potential that assistive technologies can have to help people with dementia to live at home more independently. The project was to provide a unique opportunity to test out several assistive technologies in people's homes, to seek their views on how these worked, and to assess the extent to which these technologies could adequately address their practical problems.

Background and aims of the study

ENABLE was a hypothetic-deductive study. The hypothesis was that use and usefulness of products would be dependent upon factors related to the person with dementia, their carer, the environment, the product and the research (Hagen *et al.* 2004). The research design was also exploratory/descriptive because this was the first time, in the European context, that these particular research questions were investigated (for an extensive review of the methodology see Hagen *et al.* 2004). Both quantitative and qualitative data were collected from people with dementia and their primary carers, who were predominantly family members. Their views and experiences about the respective devices installed in their homes were sought over a follow-up period. Although use and usefulness of the products were considered important primary outcome measures, the latter was also seen to be dependent on: (a) the nature of problems experienced; (b) the appropriateness of the device introduced to address these problems (such as falls at night, time disorientation); (c) the importance of the problem to the individual diagnosed with dementia and to his or her family carer.

Study inclusion and exclusion criteria

As part of the developing methodology, strict inclusion criteria were developed. Respondents were required to:

- have a diagnosis of Alzheimer's disease, vascular dementia or mixed Alzheimer's disease and vascular dementia

- have a Mini Mental State Exam (MMSE) score of 12 or above

- have a primary carer (either co-resident or living nearby)

- be aged over 50 years

- be in reasonably good nutritional and general health

- be deemed by staff to be able to benefit from one or other of these products

- provide consent to participate in the study

- live in close proximity to Dublin.

Exclusion criteria outruled those people with dementia who:

- had a major psychiatric disorder

- were involved in other drug/clinical trials

- were likely to move to long-term care within the first three months of the study.

Other 'real life' challenges in relation to the recruitment and implementation phase of this study included: the novel nature of the project; the deteriorating aspect of Alzheimer's disease and other related dementias; the natural protectiveness that many carers have for their relatives; the consent protocol which permitted people to withdraw from the study at any stage; and the desire on the researcher's part to carefully match the most appropriate device to the relevant participant.

Description of assistive technologies evaluated in Ireland

Table 8.I describes the assistive technologies evaluated in ENABLE and provides a breakdown of product distribution per person, at baseline (when devices were first installed) and at Time Four (i.e. six months after the study began). Although some people had multiple psychosocial needs, for product evaluation and so as not to confound the assessment, it was felt advisable that only one device should be supplied to each participant. The need that was most important to the person with dementia was chosen as the criterion for choosing this device. At three months, a total of 20 people had completed the study and by six months numbers had dropped to 17, representing an attrition rate of 53 per cent (n = 15) during the first six-month follow-up period. In most cases withdrawals occurred due to technical problems with the devices, due to admission to long-term care facilities, or because of difficulties adjusting to the new products. Figure 8.1 shows a pictorial description of the four assistive technologies evaluated in Ireland and described in this chapter.

Table 8.1 Description of assistive devices being tested in Ireland				
Item	Usage	Expected effect	Product distribution at baseline (N =32)	Product distribution completers to six months (N = 17)
Automatic night and day calendar	As a calendar; day, date and time of day (morning, afternoon or night) are automatically displayed.	Facilitates orientation, prevents people from going out during the night.	6	5
Item locator for lost objects	Pressing the picture of an item on a wall display panel causes the lost item to emit a warbling sound, stops when item is picked up.	Finds frequently mislaid objects such as keys, purse, etc. Reduces worries and time spent looking for mislaid objects.	11	4
Automatic night lamp	Automatic light turns on and off when the person gets in and out of bed.	Prevents falls at night, reduces anxiety.	6	3
Picture telephone	A telephone that displays pictures of nine contacts whose numbers are stored in the phone; it also has larger buttons.	Reduces anxiety surrounding the use of telephones, supports memory.	6	5

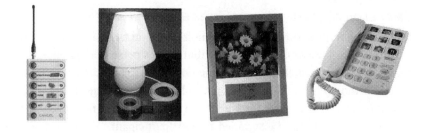

Figure 8.1: Pictorial examples of the assistive technologies evaluated in Ireland

Recruitment

People were recruited for this study from: (a) the Mercer's Institute for Research on Ageing and its National Memory Clinic; (b) Medicine for the Elderly at St James' Hospital; (c) the Old Age Psychiatry services of both St James' and St Patrick's hospital; (d) the Alzheimer Society of Ireland (ASI). Accordingly, amongst the initial 32 people recruited to the study, ten families were referred by staff from the National Memory Clinic, seven came from St Patrick's hospital, eight from the ASI, five from the Department of Medicine for the Elderly and two referrals were made by hospital-based occupational therapists. An incentive for study participation was the fact that devices would be retained free by families after study completion. However, despite this incentive and the rigorous and concerted effort used to recruit participants (including distributing information kits about products and their expected outcomes to families), a number of respondents had preconceptions about the products, causing disappointment in some cases, as products were not always what they had expected.

Respondent demographics

Table 8.2 shows the socio-demographic and cognitive characteristics for the sample of people with dementia (n = 17) who remained in the study over the first six months. Amongst the sample, 14 respondents were diagnosed with Alzheimer's disease, one had vascular dementia, and two had mixed Alzheimer's disease and vascular dementia (not shown). Most (n = 13) had a mild dementia with a median MMSE score of 22. As might be expected, there were more than twice as many women than men (12:5) in the sample. Interestingly, several of these men and women (n = 7) were continuing to live at home alone.

Table 8.2 Socio-demographic and cognitive characteristics of people with dementia (N = 17)										
Age, years		Gender		Living arrangements			MMSE		Degree of dementia	
Mean	Range	Male	Female	Alone	With spouse	With carer's family	Median	Range	Mild	Moderate
76	61–91	5	12	7	8	2	22	17	13	4

The primary carers (n = 17) had an average age of 61 years (range 36 to 81 years), five were males and 29 percent were in paid employment. Only a minority (n = 5) were in paid employment whilst continuing to provide care to their relatives. The majority received very limited formal support from government services and limited assistance from other family members (not shown).

Outcomes

As mentioned, two dependent variables, namely (a) use of products and (b) their perceived usefulness, were used to evaluate the four assistive technologies trialled in the homes of these 17 men and women with dementia who were still participating in the study at the end of six months. Questions investigating these issues were asked of both the individual and his or her primary carer at three points in time, namely three weeks, three months and six months after product installation. To check for reliability of data, the primary carer's own perception of their relative's use of the product was also investigated. Only data pertaining to Time Four are reported in this chapter. For data collected at three months see Cahill *et al.* (2007).

Person with dementia's use of product

Table 8.3 demonstrates the use of the four assistive technologies reported by people with dementia six months after their installation.

Table 8.3 Use of products reported by person with dementia six months after devices were installed (N = 17)					
Person with dementia: Have you used the product?	Type of device implemented				Total
Count	Calendar	Lamp	Locator	Telephone	
Yes	4	2	1	4	11
No	0	1	3	1	5
No answer	1	0	0	0	1
Total	5	3	4	5	17

Table 8.3 shows that according to the individual with dementia, the most frequently used ENABLE devices were the night and day calendar and the picture
telephone, where four out of five people with dementia reported they continued to use both of these devices six months after installation. As regards the
night lamp, the data show that two out of three people assessed for this device
reported they were still using it at this point in time. Less popular was the item
locator where only one out of four people with dementia reported they were
continuing to use the device six months after its installation. In total 11 out of
17 people with dementia (65%) claimed they were still using the device six
months after its installation. The positive impacts many of these assistive technologies had on the lives of these people are well illustrated in the qualitative
data:

> [I am] very satisfied, I'm very pleased with it, my little toy, it's the one thing I
> can use. I'm slow at all sorts of other things. (Man with dementia, picture
> button telephone, 61 years)

> It's very handy, it's marvellous, it saves you looking for numbers. (Woman
> with dementia, picture button telephone)

Table 8.4 Carers' perceptions of use of products by their care recipient six months after installation (N = 17)

Carer: Has person with dementia used the product?	Type of device implemented				Total
Count	Calendar	Lamp	Locator	Telephone	
Yes	4	3	0	5	12
No	0	0	3	0	3
No answer	1	0	1	0	2
Total	5	3	4	5	17

Table 8.4 shows data emerging from interviews conducted with primary
carers about their perceptions of their relatives' use of each product six months
after its installation. By and large, carers' accounts of product use tended to be
consistent with the individuals' own perceptions. Data show, for example, that
in the opinion of primary carers, the calendar, night lamp and picture telephone tended to also be used by their relative. In contrast no primary carer
reported that the item locator was now being used by their relative.

Carers' use of product

Table 8.5 reports carers' accounts of their own use of the respective products six months after their installation. Given that the products were originally designed for use by the person with dementia and not by a primary carer, the data show that in the case of both the calendar and the picture telephone these technologies were also preferred by the primary carers. For example, after six months, three out of four carers stated that they also used the night and day calendar, and four out of five claimed they used the picture telephone. Interestingly, the data demonstrate that more family carers than persons with dementia were using the item locator at this point in time.

Table 8.5 Carers' own use of assistive devices six months after installation (N = 17)					
Carer: Have you used the product?	Type of device implemented				Total
Count	Calendar	Lamp	Locator	Telephone	
Yes	3	1	2	4	10
No	1	2	1	1	5
No answer	1	0	1	0	2
Total	5	3	4	5	17

Again the qualitative data provide rich evidence of the potential such psychosocial interventions have to reduce carer burden and improve the person with dementia's self-esteem and well-being:

> I find it wonderful as sometimes my patience wears thin and I get quite stressed before we leave the house. My mother's mood was also better as she did not have to try and remember where everything was and so did not realise how forgetful she was. (Daughter carer's views about item locator)

Person with dementia's perceptions of device usefulness

Table 8.6 reports on the usefulness of the respective devices from the perspective of the sample of people with dementia. Data show how 12 out of 17 people with dementia (70%) reported the installed technologies were still in their view useful for them six months after their installation. There were only three cases where respondents had difficulty understanding the question and were unable to answer it. One person supplied with an item locator reported that it was not useful and in another case a woman who had a picture telephone installed also denied that it was useful.

Table 8.6 People with dementia – usefulness of assistive devices six months after installation (N = 17)

Person with dementia: Is the product useful?	Type of device implemented				Total
Count	Calendar	Lamp	Locator	Telephone	
Yes	4	2	2	4	12
No	0	1	0	1	2
No answer	1	0	2	0	3
Total	5	3	4	5	17

Carers' perceptions of usefulness of device

When carers' own views were sought about the respective usefulness of these devices, data show that 13 out of 17 (76%) reported that they thought the device with which they were supplied was useful (see Table 8.7).

Table 8.7 shows that in relation to the night lamp and telephone each of the primary carers when interviewed reported that these devices were useful. Some technical problems with the item locator resulted in two carers stating they were unable to report on its usefulness and one other carer claimed it was not useful.

Table 8.7 Carers' perceptions of usefulness of assistive devices for person with dementia six months after installation (N = 17)

Carer: Is the device useful for person with dementia?	Type of device implemented				Total
Count	Calendar	Lamp	Locator	Telephone	
Yes	4	3	1	5	13
No	0	0	1	0	1
No answer	1	0	2	0	3
Total	5	3	4	5	17

Case studies

Whilst quantitative and qualitative data provide preliminary evidence of the benefits that most of these newly installed assistive technologies had on the lives of people in this study, the data fail to capture the realities and complexities of these families' everyday lives, their fears, frustrations and anxieties experienced whilst coping with a dementia and coming to terms with such psychosocial interventions. Therefore, to gain more valid portrayals (Patton 1990) and to understand in more detail the unique problems the sample was experiencing, the section below details three case studies from the research. The case studies yield subjective insights into the psychosocial worlds of these men and women and illustrate the potential that assistive technologies have to address some of the practical problems that persons with dementia may experience and the reasons why in some cases technologies failed to work.

Case example – Ernest

Ernest was a 69-year-old Dubliner, diagnosed with mixed Alzheimer's disease and vascular dementia. Aware of his diagnosis, he was enthused about ENABLE from its commencement, was willing to talk openly about his illness and excited that he was going to receive a new 'helping aid'. His wife, Vera, reported that one of his main problems was that he was disorientated in time and would often get up during the night, making his way to the kitchen to have breakfast. Rather than argue with him, she tended to allow him do this and usually later persuaded him to return to bed. She was keen to get support and stated that her husband's night wakefulness was disruptive to her own sleep. The automatic night and day calendar was seen to have the most potential for Ernest and his wife. Despite his enthusiasm for ENABLE, initially the unfamiliarity of the design of the night and day calendar, combined with his failing eyesight, made adapting to this new intervention more difficult for him than had been previously planned. It took him longer to read the text on the calendar and yet he refused Vera's assistance, determined to read the text himself.

After six months, Vera reported that the night and day calendar had been very effective. She recalled that one particular night her husband woke and rather than ask her what time it was, he went to the calendar independently, clarified from the calendar, which was illuminated, that it was still night and returned to bed. Another morning she said he rose shortly after five, and despite her protests, he went down for breakfast as the 'calendar had said it was morning' (the calendar switches automatically to display morning at 5 am). Another unexpected benefit of the night and day calendar for Ernest was the fact that he attended a day centre where each day, staff tended to talk clients through the days of the week, by way of helping to orientate them. Ernest felt very pleased that, as a result of the night and day calendar, he now always knew in advance which day of the week it was, and indeed told his friends at the day centre about the product. When interviewed, Ernest reported that he used the calendar and found it very useful. He said the device gave him greater independence and lessened his dependence on his wife. The technology was also helpful to Vera as her husband no longer repeatedly asked questions about the days of the week or the time of day. In the past, she had found this particularly stressful. Overall, Vera reported that her husband had become more independent and was coping much better because of the device – 'because it helps him, otherwise the days would pass and he wouldn't know, he looks at this (the calendar) and he knows where he is'.

Case example – Sarah

When Sarah first became involved with ENABLE, she was 69 years old and lived with her bachelor son in Dublin. Her daughter, the primary carer who was the main informant for the project, lived close by. Sarah was referred to ENABLE because she often mislaid items around the house and at times blamed others in the house, particularly her son who lived with her, for losing her things. Her son mentioned that when his mother behaved in this accusatory manner he reacted negatively and as a result their relationship had deteriorated over recent times. In turn Sarah reported that she often felt frustrated with her son when he did things without telling her. In view of her short-term memory loss and capacity for mislaying things around the house, it was decided that the item locator might be a potentially useful assistive technology to help address Sarah's difficulty.

Initially Sarah thought that the item locator would be an ideal device for her, and her children also supported its implementation, recognising its potential. However, from the implementation phase, there were problems. First, the installation of the device was delayed due to technical problems and all item locators had to be recalled. This meant that the family were waiting longer for the device than was previously expected. Despite these delays, Sarah and her family remained positive and motivated. However, once the replacement device was successfully implemented, technical problems persisted. As an example, Sarah had difficulty hearing the tags: 'The locator did not work as we could not hear it' (respondent diary entry, carer/daughter). In addition, there were times when the device failed to ring, which resulted in it not being used at all. Eventually, the carer reported that the item locator was causing her mother more confusion than help and the family reluctantly withdrew from the study. This case study points to the importance of designing and implementing devices that have undergone extensive and rigorous pre-testing to avoid expectations people might have from being unfulfilled. The case study also highlights the importance of thorough and ongoing needs assessment in all cases where someone with a dementia is being assessed for an assistive device.

Case example – Gordon

Gordon, aged 59 years, was the youngest participant in ENABLE. He lived with his wife, Kate, and three children (whose ages ranged from 2 to 16 years) in a quiet housing estate outside Dublin. The family had recently moved home from a two-storey house to a bungalow to facilitate Gordon's mobility problems. Since being diagnosed with Alzheimer's disease, Gordon had resigned from his job and was now spending most of his time at home alone, as his wife worked part-time and his children were either at school or attending a childminder. Kate mentioned that the house move and loss of a second income had caused her worry and some financial strain. Other practical problems encountered daily by Gordon included short-term memory loss, instability of gait and social isolation. New learning was also a challenge for him, as he tended to be frightened of trying new things out in case he failed. He was also frustrated that he was no longer able to do many of the routine tasks he previously found easy. Gordon was a very sociable person who, throughout his life, always had a large social network, but now due to his diagnosis and having to take early retirement he felt socially isolated. For this reason, the picture button telephone was thought to be an appropriate intervention as it was hoped this would help keep him in touch with relatives and friends. He had previously tried other communication devices such as mobile phones but found they were unsuitable for his needs. It was hoped that the introduction of the picture button telephone would boost his self-esteem and improve his ability to communicate with others.

Gordon went through some obvious changes during the ENABLE trial. At assessment he seemed very low: 'I don't enjoy anything anymore…I worry all the time…nothing makes me happy anymore.' However, as the project progressed, his mood clearly changed: 'I wasn't content at the start of this, I used to go to the park and cry but that didn't solve anything, it just made it worse, now I'm coming around' (Time Three). Of all ENABLE participants, Gordon was most open about discussing his illness and experiences and was also actively involved in his health care decisions. As the ENABLE trial progressed, Gordon began showing signs of accepting and dealing better with his diagnosis, using the picture telephone, and implementing coping mechanisms, including attending a day centre and going back to his local pub for a pint. However, despite these positive adjustments, Kate began to find the caregiver role (including child care) combined with working part-time and running the household increasingly more challenging and eventually she chose to take a career break. The case study demonstrates the differing needs and aspirations of a person and their carer; that is, on the one hand data show that over the period during which the picture telephone had been installed Gordon gained independence and learned to do more things for himself. However, despite these small victories, during the same time period, Kate began to feel the pressure of caring more acutely. Both spoke very positively about the picture telephone, how useful it was and how much they enjoyed using it.

Discussion and conclusion

The Irish experience with ENABLE has shown that including people with a mild to moderate dementia and their primary carers in longitudinal research was feasible. Most participants, despite their cognitive deficits, were competent at understanding and answering all questions asked of them and in certain cases several could provide rich descriptive information about the impact these psychosocial interventions had on their lives. In the majority of cases, there was also a degree of consistency between what the primary carer reported about the use of the product and the individual's own experience. The Irish experience suggests that including people with dementia in a study of this kind is empowering. The approach taken helped to motivate people to use the devices, as participants were involved from the very inception of the project in matters that directly affected them and their daily routines.

Our findings show that the majority of participants (65%) equipped with ENABLE products were still using the devices six months after their installation and most people found them useful. Likewise, a large majority of family carers (70%) reported their relative used the device and most of these family carers themselves also found the products useful six months after installation. Overall, our results support the hypothesis that the use and usefulness of assistive technology can be explained by factors relating to the person with dementia, the carer, the environment, the researcher and the product itself. Findings showed that the ability to use products was influenced by whether a cognitively impaired person could remember how to operate the device, whether that person was familiar with its design and whether the device was reliable and worked efficiently.

Several technical problems with the ENABLE products were witnessed within the first few months of the project being launched. However, most of these problems were easily resolved. Other technical problems persisted (for example, in the case of the item locator and the night lamp), which meant that products were not always reliable for the individual or the family carer. Hence findings about their use and usefulness may have been influenced by inefficiencies in their performance. In interpreting the results from this study these issues need to be seriously considered since inevitably they may well have affected attrition rates, individual attitudes to and assessment of products.

Overall our recommendations on the basis of the ENABLE assessment study in Ireland are as follows:

- Ensure that prototype products are more fully refined and pre-tested with a sample of cognitively intact older people, before in-home implementation studies are developed with persons with dementia.

- Each ENABLE product has potential application for people who do not have dementia. Research on the acceptability of assistive technology to older people in general reflects a complex model that gives rise to tensions in acceptability (McCreadie and Tinker 2005). The future commercial availability of these devices will need to take these findings into consideration. However, given this, wider availability to cognitively intact older people might also enhance their acceptability and utility as memory aids for older people who then go on to develop a dementia.

- The ENABLE project has highlighted the need to develop relevant social policy responses to the issue of assistive technology for people with dementia in Ireland.

Finally, our experience in ENABLE raises several critical questions about the role of service providers in relation to the assessment of people with dementia for assistive technology; the in-home installation of these technologies; their cost; and their maintenance and monitoring (see Cahill *et al.* 2007). Issues to be resolved include:

- Which professional group should assess people with dementia for assistive technologies, and in the context of scarce resources, on what basis should client need be determined?

- From where should technologies be supplied (i.e. hospital departments, day care centres, disability resource centres or community services)?

- Should occupational therapists, community social workers, public health nurses, community mental health nurses or staff from Alzheimer's societies install these technologies?

- How can respective costs for technologies be met (i.e. should they be freely available, as in the case of some Scandinavian countries, or should a small user payment be levied)?

- How can local engineers be motivated to take a more active interest in the area of designing and refining technologies?

- Should devices be loaned to people for a designated period of time, given that their usefulness will inevitably diminish over time?

These are all practical and relevant questions that should now enter debates on in-home implementation of assistive devices for people with dementia and family carers. They are also issues that need to be kept alive and brought to the attention of policymakers, planners and those involved in the development and delivery of educational courses directed at upskilling professionals involved in dementia care.

References

Bjørneby, S., Topo, P. and Holthe, T. (eds) (1999) *TED. Technology, Ethics and Dementia. A Guidebook on How to Apply Technology in Dementia Care.* Oslo: Norwegian Centre for Dementia Care, INFO-banken.

Cahill, S., Begley, E., Faulkner, J.P. and Hagen, I. (2007) '"It gives me a sense of independence": findings from Ireland on the use and usefulness of assistive technologies for people with dementia.' *Technology and Disability 19*, 133–142.

Ferri, C., Prince, M., Brayne, C., Brodaty, H., *et al.* (2005) 'Global prevalence of dementia: a delphi, consensus study.' *The Lancet 366*, 2112–2117.

Gallagher, C. (2006) 'Social Policy and a Good Life in Old Age.' In E. O'Dell (ed.) *Older People in Modern Ireland.* Dublin: Johnswood Press.

Hagen, I., Holthe, T., Gilliard, J., Topo, P., *et al.* (2004) 'Development of a protocol for the assessment of assistive aids for people with dementia.' *Dementia: The International Journal of Social Research and Practice 3*, 3, 263–281.

Holthe, T., Hagen, I. and Bjorneby, S. (1999) 'What day is it today? Using an automatic calendar.' *Journal of Dementia Care 7*, 4, 26–27.

Marshall, M. (ed.) (2000) *ASTRID: A Social Technological Response to Meeting the Needs of Individuals with Dementia and their Carers.* London: Hawker Publications.

McCreadie, C. and Tinker, A. (2005) 'The acceptability of assistive technology to older people.' *Ageing & Society 25*, 91–110.

O'Shea, E. (2006) 'Public Policy for Dependent Older People in Ireland: Review and Reform.' In E. O'Dell (ed.) *Older People in Modern Ireland.* Dublin: Johnswood Press.

O'Shea, E. and O'Reilly, S. (1999a) *An Action Plan for Dementia.* Dublin: National Council on Ageing and Older People.

O'Shea, E. and O'Reilly, S. (1999b) *The Economic and Social Costs of Alzheimer's Disease and Related Dementias in Ireland: An Aggregate Analysis.* Working Paper no. 25. Galway: National University of Ireland, Department of Economics.

Patton, M. (1990) *Qualitative Evaluation and Research Methods.* Newbury Park: Sage.

Sweep, M.A.J. (1998) *Technology for People with Dementia: User Requirements.* Eindhoven, the Netherlands: Institute for Gerontechnology, University of Technology.

Wimo, A., Jonsson, L. and Winblad, B. (2006) 'An estimate of the worldwide prevalence and direct costs of dementia in 2003.' *Dementia and Geriatric Cognitive Disorders 21*, 175–181.

Woolham, J. (2006) *Safe at Home. The Effectiveness of Assistive Technology in Supporting the Independence of People with Dementia.* London: Hawker Publications.

Woolham, J., Frisby, B., Quinn, S., Smart, W. and Moore, A. (2002) *The Safe at Home Project.* London: Hawker Publications.

Further reading and related references

Bjørneby, S., Topo, P., Cahill, S., Begley, E., *et al.* (2004) 'Ethical considerations in the ENABLE project.' *Dementia 3*, 3, 297–312.

Cahill, S., Begley, E., Topo, P., Saarikalle, K., *et al.* (2004) '"I know where this is going and I know it won't go back": hearing the individual's voice in dementia quality of life assessments.' *Dementia 3*, 3, 313–330.

Chapman, A. (2001) 'There's no place like a smart home.' *Journal of Dementia Care 9*, 1, 28–31.

Chapman, A. (2001) 'A smarter system is always at hand.' *Journal of Dementia Care 9*, 2, 8.

Duff, P. and Cullen, K. (1999) 'Assistive technology: new opportunities for people with dementia and their carers.' Paper presented to International Conference on Ageing 'Promoting Independence and Quality of Life for Older Persons'. Arlington, VA.

Gilliard, J. and Hagen, I. (eds) (2004) Enabling Technologies for People with Dementia: Cross-national Analysis Report. WP 4.5/Deliverable no. 4.5.1. Project funded by the European Commission under the 'Quality of Life and Management of Living Resources' under the Framework Programme 5. Available at www.dementia-voice.org.uk/Projects/EnableFinalProject.pdf, accessed 7 August 2008.

Kinney, J.M., Kart, C.S., Murdoch, L.D. and Conley, C.J. (2004) 'Striving to provide safety assistance for families of elders: the SAFE House project.' *Dementia 3*, 3, 351–370.

Marshall, M. (2002) 'Technology and technophobia.' *Journal of Dementia Care 10*, 5, 14–15.

Marshall, M. (2003) 'Not just because we can do it.' *Journal of Dementia Care 11*, 6, 10.

Marshall, M., Duff, P. and Cullen, K. (2000) 'ASTRID: introducing assistive technology.' *Journal of Dementia Care 8*, 4, 18–19.

Topo, P., Maki, O., Saarikalle, K., Clarke, N., *et al.* (2004) 'Assessment of a music-based multimedia program for people with dementia.' *Dementia: The International Journal of Social Research and Practice 3*, 3.

Useful websites

www.astridguide.org, accessed 7 August 2008
www.enableproject.org, accessed 7 August 2008

ENABLE partners

Bath Institute of Medical Engineering: www.bath.ac.uk/bime, accessed 7 August 2008
Dementia Services Information and Development Centre: dsidc@stjames.ie
Dementia Voice: office@dementia-voice.org.uk
Inger Hagen, scientific co-ordinator: post@ihagen.no
Norwegian Centre for Dementia Research: knut.engedal@nordemens.no
Sidsel Bjørneby: sibjoern@online.no
STAKES – National Research and Development Centre for Health and Welfare: paivi.topo@stakes.fi
Work Research Centre: p.duff@wrc-research.ie

PART III

Psychological, Emotional and Social Support

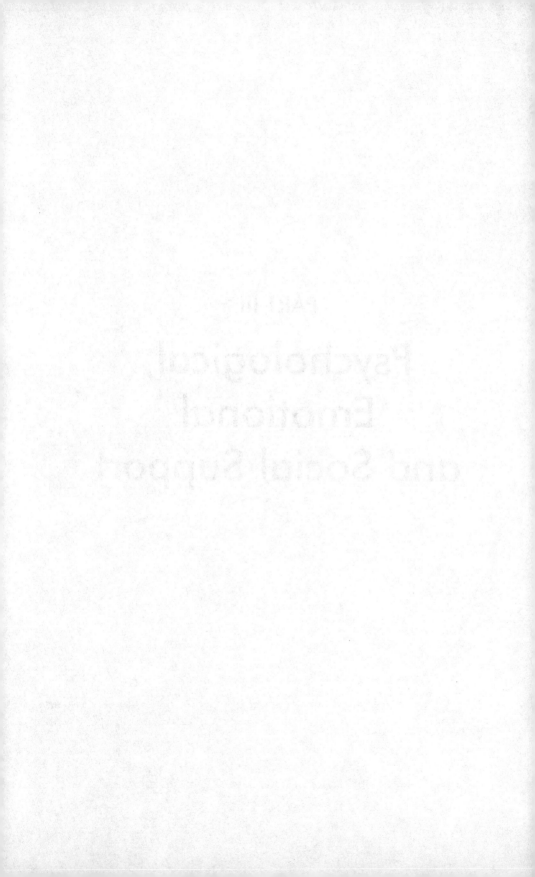

Chapter 9

Group Psychotherapy for People with Early Dementia

Richard Cheston

Overview

Supporting and meeting the emotional needs of people with dementia are now recognised as important aims for health and social care professionals. This is reflected in the increasing use of psychotherapy and counselling techniques over the last ten years. The most widespread means of using psychotherapeutic intervention with people with dementia is probably through group work. This is particularly beneficial in that it can create a sense of shared experience and provide a safe environment for people to explore their internal world. Issues in setting up a group are discussed in this chapter with particular reference to the Dementia Voice Group Psychotherapy Project. Analysis of data collected provided significant evidence for a treatment effect, lowering both anxiety and depression in the group participants. In addition, a case study is provided which highlights the way that group work can help people with dementia 'come to terms' with their diagnosis.

Psychotherapeutic group work with older people with a cognitive impairment has been described since the early 1950s. However, it is only since person-centred forms of care have become firmly established over the last 10 to 15 years in the UK that this form of providing emotional support for people with dementia has begun to develop. Yet, while there has been increasing interest in using psychotherapy and counselling skills with people with dementia, relatively few studies have systematically explored the effectiveness of this work. It still remains unclear, therefore, which form or forms of psychotherapy – whether group or individual work, directive or non-directive, educational or exploratory approaches – constitute the most effective intervention.

One of the earliest developments of psychotherapeutic approaches with people with dementia was that of 'Validation therapy' (Feil 1990, 1992, 1993). Feil suggested that in many cases neurological damage interacted with unresolved issues from a person's past so that those psychological defences that had been used up to that point were no longer effective. She suggested that this precipitated the person with dementia returning to the past in order to work through these unresolved issues. Consequently the task of the Validation therapist was to validate or support this inward journey back through time. In order to do this, Feil stressed the importance of therapists listening with empathy, using non-threatening questions in order to build up trust and not confronting people with the loss of their abilities.

Feil's work has proved to be influential – in part because she was one of the earliest voices urging dementia care workers to take the emotional needs of people with dementia seriously. Yet, two criticisms can be made of this way of working. First, there is the danger that in associating the apparent confusion of some older people with unresolved psychological issues, we risk attributing the presence of dementia to personal, rather than organic factors. Second, although we are all influenced by our past, there is a danger that in looking backwards we obscure the current reality for people with dementia. Arguably the most important psychological task for group therapists is one of helping people to resolve current rather than past issues in their lives.

Person-centred care and group psychotherapy

A wide range of individual psychotherapeutic work with people with dementia has been described including psychodynamic (e.g. Sinason 1992), cognitive behavioural (e.g. Scholey and Woods 2003; Teri and Gallagher-Thomson 1991) and humanistic (e.g. Bryden 2002; Stokes and Goudie 1990). An evidence base for individual psychotherapy is also beginning to emerge (e.g. Burns *et al.* 2005).

Despite the increasing popularity of individual forms of therapy, probably the single most common means of using psychotherapy as a way of intervening with people with dementia has been through group work. The review by Cheston (1998a), for instance, identified over twice as many reports of groups compared to work with individuals. However, this review went on to point out that despite the increase in this form of clinical work, there was little if any substantive research evidence relating to its effectiveness.

Nevertheless, regardless of the lack of an available evidence base, the need to provide psychotherapy and counselling for people with dementia is becoming ever more apparent. This is partly because the introduction of new medication designed to enhance levels of cognitive functioning has increased the numbers of people with suspected Alzheimer's disease who are presenting themselves for assessment and diagnosis at an earlier stage. This in turn has led to the need to provide support to enable people with dementia to grieve for their losses and to begin the process of learning to adjust to the changes that can come with living with dementia.

Thus, an English government document *Everybody's Business* (Department of Health 2005) has provided guidelines for local commissioners of services to use when establishing memory assessment services. Its recommendations include the need for pre- and post-diagnostic counselling, as well as explaining the diagnosis to the person with dementia and giving information about their prognosis and their care options.

Within this context, group work provides a number of therapeutic advantages over individual counselling. In particular, by bringing together people who might otherwise be dealing with such significant changes in isolation, it is possible to help develop a sense that experiences are shared. This desire to create a supportive context for people to talk about what was happening to them was stimulated by the publication of a book by Robyn Yale (1995) setting out how to establish, run and evaluate support groups for people with dementia.

Yet, just as there are an enormous variety of individual forms of psychotherapy, so group therapists can be influenced by a wide range of therapeutic orientations. Broadly speaking, groups for people with dementia tend to reflect two different strands of work:

1. *Educational groups.* The emphasis is to teach people about their illness and to encourage them to use a variety of strategies in order to facilitate adjustment to their impairments such as talks from visiting speakers (e.g. McAfee *et al.* 1989), information about Alzheimer's disease (e.g. Haggerty 1990) and teaching memory strategies (e.g. see Chapter 7 of this book; Thrower 1998).

2. *Emotionally focused groups.* The emphasis is upon helping people to share their experiences with others. Arguably, one of the most important aspects of a support group is to enable group participants to feel listened to, and to feel that their experience of dementia is important. In addition to the process of talking and sharing experiences, a variety of potentially therapeutic interventions can be employed including anxiety management skills (e.g. Marshall 2001),

focusing on relationship issues (e.g. Hawkins and Eagger 1999) and how to cope with the loss of independence (e.g. Barton *et al.* 2001).

General issues in setting up a group

When thinking about establishing a group, a variety of issues needs to be considered:

- psychological mindedness
- locating groups within a service
- co-working
- involving carers in the work.

Psychological mindedness

Decisions about who should be involved in a group are related to a wealth of considerations, including the context in which the group is established and its overall aims. Where, however, the aim of the group is to share experiences, then it is important to look at the capacity of potential participants to be involved in such work – in part this relates to their ability to communicate effectively, for instance, their cognitive level, their verbal fluency and the presence of any sensory loss. Perhaps of at least equal significance is the *psychological mindedness* of group members – their ability to think about their internal world.

My own experiences have increasingly led me to think about the importance of individuals' personal resources prior to their developing cognitive problems. Some people (although by no means all) who have considerable difficulties in thinking about what has happened to them might be described as having had a rather fragile pre-morbid personality: that is to say they seem to have been people who presented to the world an idea of themselves as a person without imperfections, like a porcelain vase. Like the vase, their view of themselves was of a beautiful thing, but also delicate and easily fractured. As such my sense is sometimes that these people, who cannot now acknowledge in public that their memory has become flawed, also found it hard before their illness to acknowledge imperfections in their way of being. Instead their concern was to preserve their personal authority and prestige. Now, when they are confronted with a gradual decline in their intellectual abilities, their tendency is, once again, to ignore or to dismiss this evidence.

Although groups can be places that are able to tolerate many ways of managing and thinking (or not thinking) about life, it will be important to consider the balance of such methods of coping that participants to a group bring. The best groups tend to have a balance between people who are inclined to think (but risk being overwhelmed) and people who prefer to act (but risk ignoring what is happening).

Locating groups within a service

Many clinical services will not be familiar with either the demands or the needs of group work. At times this may lead to a lack of referrals or to the necessary boundaries around groups being compromised. It is important then for groups to be firmly established within the consciousness of services, and to be seen to meet a clear service need. The service as a whole should value the role that groups can play and permit the groups to function. In practical terms, then, a valued place within a service would allow adequate transport for group members, rooms for the group to meet and to assemble in without interruption or interference, and a working space that is potentially therapeutic.

Co-working

Group work is often seen to require joint facilitators, and this in turn necessitates a shared model of working and either shared supervision or a clear agreement about peer supervision. Therapists cannot work together without both the capacity for reflective thinking and opportunities to reflect together on the work.

Involving carers in the work

Just as there is a wide range of therapeutic orientations for group work, so there is a continuum along which carers may be involved. Where the purpose of the group is to provide a context in which participants can explore their experiences in a safe and containing manner, then the intrusion of carers into the therapeutic space needs to be avoided. At the same time, if the group is to be successful, then carers as much as participants need to have a commitment to the group.

Alternatively, if the aim of the group is to provide a supportive educational framework, then the role of carers becomes stronger. In the supportive seminar model of working (Snyder *et al.* 1995), carers accompany group participants to the first session. After they have met one another, one facilitator can meet with the carers and the other can begin the group with the participants. Each group can look at what people would like to get out of the group, and to think about the worst aspect of having a memory problem. At the end of the session, the two groups can come back together to share their thoughts.

The Dementia Voice Group Psychotherapy project (the DVGP)

Due to the absence of methodologically appropriate studies exploring the impact of group psychotherapy, the DVGP set out to evaluate the impact of a ten-week intervention on participants' levels of depression and anxiety compared to a baseline period and follow-up. The project involved establishing six psychotherapy groups across the south-west of England for people who had been diagnosed with Alzheimer's disease or another form of dementia. It was funded by grants from the Mental Health Foundation and from Avon and Wiltshire Mental Health Partnership Trust. Each group lasted for ten weeks and was facilitated by the author in collaboration with either one or two co-facilitators who varied from group to group.

Participants

In all 42 people took part in the groups, all of whom were assessed as having either a mild or a moderate level of dementia. Most people lived at home with their husband or wife, although some lived on their own or in nursing homes. All of the participants had a Mini Mental State Exam (MMSE) score of 18 or above, indicating that they had a mild or moderate level of cognitive impairment.

Therapeutic aims

The central aim of these groups was to bring people with dementia together to talk about 'what it's like when your memory doesn't work as well as it used to do'. Participants were encouraged to share their experiences with each other and to discuss the emotional impact of these experiences on them.

The need to listen and bear witness

The groups in this project focused upon the experiences of participants in the here and now, and upon the impact of these experiences upon relationships, including those formed within the matrix of the group. The task for group participants was to think about 'what it's like when your memory isn't as good as it used to be'. The task of the group therapists was to facilitate this process of reflection by interpreting material that was brought to the group in terms of its underlying emotional significance and within the context of the group processes. As such this approach differs markedly from other therapeutic forms of work with people with dementia such as Validation Therapy, Life-review Therapy (e.g. Garland 1994) or Reminiscence Therapy (e.g. Bender 1994). A fuller description of the use of this style of working within a group setting with people with dementia can be found elsewhere (Cheston 1998b; Cheston and Jones 2002; Cheston, Jones and Gilliard 2003a).

Analysis of results

Participants and their carers were interviewed at four different points: about six weeks before the groups started; at the start of the groups; at the end of the groups; and ten weeks after the groups had finished. Twenty-seven people finished the groups and the follow-up period, and baseline data were available from 19 of these participants. Tape recordings of one of the groups were also made to enable a more detailed examination of the process of change occurring within the groups.

Changes in levels of depression and anxiety

Data was collected independently of the facilitators by a research officer for Dementia Voice (Kerry Jones). Statistical analysis of the data from those 19 participants who completed all three phases of the project provided significant evidence for a treatment effect lowering levels of both anxiety and depression. This change was maintained at follow-up. For the eight participants who joined at the start of the intervention phase, there was evidence of a significant fall in levels of anxiety but not depression. In addition, significantly more group members showed evidence of reliable change in levels of depression during the intervention period compared to either the baseline or the follow-up periods (Cheston et al. 2003b).

Case example – Robert – changes in awareness

Although it is important to establish the impact of the groups on levels of anxiety and depression, of equal importance is the way in which individuals within the group gradually 'came to terms' with their diagnosis. In psychotherapeutic terms, this growth of awareness can be viewed as a process in which difficult experiences or thoughts are first of all pushed away, and then gradually worked through. As an individual becomes aware of these problematic experiences, so their level of anxiety or distress initially increases but then subsides as the experiences become gradually assimilated into their existing patterns of awareness.

Watkins et al. (2006) have analysed tape recordings from the ten sessions over which a different group ran. They focused on the changes in awareness shown as the group progressed by one group participant, Robert. During the first session Robert defined his problem as a selective loss of short-term memory that did not affect other areas of his life. He referred to other people that he knew at a club that he attended, saying that 'half of them have got Alzheimer's or something near'. Watkins *et al.* (2006) suggest that during this session he was in a position of warding off awareness of both his diagnostic status and the implications of this.

Without doubt the pivotal session for Robert individually, and perhaps collectively for the group as a whole, was session four. In this session, a series of participants in the group responded to Robert's challenge ('I don't think that anyone here has Alzheimer's disease') by asserting not only that they did have Alzheimer's disease but that they felt frightened, guilty or ashamed at the knowledge. Whereas before this session Robert had not acknowledged that he had Alzheimer's disease, after it he never again denied that he did have the disease. An example of this change in Robert's accounting for his memory problems was shown in session seven in which he joked about having had the results from a computerised tomography (CT) scan fed back to him:

Robert: I got the results back yesterday and it said that my brain had shrunk very, very slightly in the cavity, which is fairly symptomatic of the onset of Alzheimer's. And so I asked, 'If it's the *onset*, what happens when you're there' [group laughs]… and he said, 'Very little more' [laughter]. I mean if you get to the point where you couldn't remember anything at all then the brain wouldn't have got any smaller but it's this shrinkage that brings about this symptom of short-term memory loss, which is quite intriguing. So I'm not particularly bothered by it, but it was interesting to go through it.

In the ninth session Robert reflected upon how he had changed over the course of the group:

Robert: I don't see the problem now the way, the problem of declining memory, the way I did before…

Janet: You didn't accept it then before?

Robert: Well I did accept it but it frightened me. But I thought, well, I'm going mad, I'm going crazy. I thought what am I going to be like in another five years?

In the complex mesh of emotional states that surround a problematic experience such as a diagnosis of having Alzheimer's disease, it is possible to distinguish between primary emotions caused by the experience itself (e.g. loss, grief, rage, fear) and secondary emotions that involve an indirect response to these primary emotions. One of the most significant of these secondary responses is that of shame – for instance, in the reaction that it is shameful to be weak and that displaying one's emotions is embarrassing. It is often these secondary emotions that inhibit the emotional processing of the problematic material and which prevent the material from being properly assimilated into existing schemata. In this regard it is particularly interesting that prominent in the discussions in week four was the acknowledgement by many participants of their emotional unease about the diagnosis. For instance, one participant (Jenny) talked about her dread that she would become '*useless*, you know. Not having all my faculties'.

Watkins *et al.* (2006) suggested that in addressing these secondary emotions the group facilitated the processing of the primary emotions by participants. It may be that the group achieves much of its therapeutic potency through, in Yalom's terms (1970), a sense of universality – that the shared nature of this condition means that to have Alzheimer's disease is not shameful, and that to express one's distress in a safe and containing environment is not embarrassing.

Conclusion

Although research evidence is only just beginning to emerge to support the use of psychotherapeutic group work with people with dementia, there are important signs that this form of work can enable group participants to work through some of the emotional consequences that dementia brings with it. As group participants work through some of these issues, so they can feel that they are not alone and thus that their position is not hopeless. Consequently, as Cheston *et al.* (2003b) suggest, there is evidence that levels of anxiety and depression may reduce.

Yet the evidence base for psychotherapy with people with dementia is only just beginning to emerge and several caveats are important: first, not all people with dementia will be suitable for, or may benefit from, group work; second, the nature of group work can vary enormously, and not all forms of group work may be therapeutic. Interestingly, an as yet unpublished small-scale study that I have led has compared a directive and structured educational group with the sort of group used during the DVGP. Although the number of people in each arm of this study was small (only eight people received each intervention), those in the exploratory groups showed similar levels of improvement in their levels of depression and anxiety, while those in the educational groups became worse. One of the crucial differences in the exploratory and directive groups was that in the latter there was much less opportunity to make sense out of their own feelings, and instead participants were provided with a much greater level of information, possibly before they were ready to manage it adequately.

The central element of group work, then, may well be the opportunity to offer people time and space to think about themselves in the context of other people: other people both similar and dissimilar to themselves. The process of meeting others in a similar position brings both hope and threat: hope because to experience others in a similar position is to have a sense of not being on one's own; threat because this process is one in which change can be made real. A central task for group facilitators is to manage the tensions within the group as participants deal with these themes of hope and threat. In doing so, the group alternates between approaching and avoiding the nature of their similarity.

A fundamental aim of group work is to provide a safe environment in which participants are able to explore their own emotional world. These groups provided a setting in which people can gain a sense that they have not been forgotten, that they will be remembered, that what has happened has been important. As one group member said: 'Just because I've got a failing memory, doesn't mean that I'm a failure.'

References

Barton, J., Piney, C., Berg, M. and Parker, C. (2001) 'Coping with forgetfulness group.' *Newsletter of the Psychologists' Special Interest Group in the Elderly 77*, 19–25.

Bender, M. (1994) 'An Interesting Confusion: What Can We Do with Reminiscence Groupwork?' In J. Bornat (ed.) *Reminiscence Reviewed: Perspectives, Evaluations, Achievements*. Maidenhead: Open University Press.

Bryden, C. (2002) 'A person-centred approach to counselling, psychotherapy and rehabilitation of people diagnosed with dementia in the early stages.' *Dementia 1*, 141–156.

Burnham, M. (2008) 'Memory Group Rehabilitation for People with Early Stage Dementia.' In E. Moniz-Cook and J. Manthorpe (eds) *Psychosocial Interventions in Early Dementia: Evidence-Based Practice*. London: Jessica Kingsley Publishers.

Burns, A., Guthrie, E., Marino-Francis, F., Busby, C., *et al*. (2005) 'Brief psychotherapy in Alzheimer's disease: a randomised controlled trial.' *British Journal of Psychiatry 187*, 143–147.

Cheston, R. (1998a) 'Psychotherapy and dementia: a review of the literature.' *British Journal of Medical Psychology 71*, 211–231.

Cheston, R. (1998b) 'Psychotherapeutic work with dementia sufferers.' *Social Work Practice 12*, 199–207.

Cheston, R. and Jones, K. (2002) 'A Place to Work It All Out Together.' In S. Benson (ed.) *Dementia Topics for the Millenium and Beyond*. London: Hawker Publications.

Cheston, R., Jones, K. and Gilliard, J. (2003a) 'Remembering and Forgetting: Group Work with People Who Have Dementia.' In T. Adams and J. Manthorpe (eds) *Dementia Care*. London: Edward Arnold.

Cheston, R., Jones, K. and Gilliard, J. (2003b) 'Group psychotherapy and people with dementia.' *Aging and Mental Health 7*, 452–461.

Department of Health (2005) *Everybody's Business*. London: The Stationery Office (see www.dh.gov.uk, accessed 8 August 2008).

Feil, N. (1990) *Validation: The Feil Method*. Cleveland, OH: Edward Feil Productions.

Feil, N. (1992) 'Validation therapy.' *Geriatric Nursing* May/June, 129–133.

Feil, N. (1993) *The Validation Breakthrough: Simple Techniques for Communicating with Alzheimer's-type Dementia*. Baltimore, MA: Health Promotions Inc.

Garland, J. (1994) 'What Splendour, It All Coheres: Life-review Therapy with Older People.' In J. Bornat (ed.) *Reminiscence Reviewed: Perspectives, Evaluations, Achievements*. Maidenhead: Open University Press.

Haggerty, A. (1990) 'Psychotherapy for patients with Alzheimer's disease.' *Advances 7*, 55–60.

Hawkins, D. and Eagger, S. (1999) 'Group therapy: sharing the pain of the diagnosis.' *Journal of Dementia Care 6, 5*, 12–14.

McAfee, M., Ruhl, P., Bell, P. and Martichuski, D. (1989) 'Including persons with early stage Alzheimer's disease in support groups and strategy planning.' *The American Journal of Alzheimer's Disease and Related Disorders and Research*, Nov/Dec, 18–22.

Marshall, A. (2001) 'Coping in early dementia: the findings of a new type of support group.' Unpublished PhD thesis, University of Surrey.

Scholey, K. and Woods, R.T. (2003) 'A series of brief cognitive therapy interventions with people experiencing both dementia and depression: a description of techniques and common themes.' *Clinical Psychology and Psychotherapy 10*, 175–185.

Sinason, V. (1992) *Mental Handicap and the Human Condition*. London: Free Association Books.

Snyder, L., Quayhagen, M.P., Sheperd, S. and Bower, D. (1995) 'Supportive seminar groups: an intervention for early stage dementia patients.' *Gerontologist 35*, 691–695.

Stokes, G. and Goudie, F. (1990) 'Counselling Confused Elderly People.' In G. Stokes and F. Goudie (eds) *Working with People with Dementia*. Bicester: Winslow.

Teri, L. and Gallagher-Thomson, D. (1991) 'Cognitive-behavioural interventions for treatment of depression in Alzheimer's patients.' *Gerontologist 31*, 413–416.

Thrower, C. (1998) 'Support and a crucial sense of belonging.' *Journal of Dementia Care 6*, 3, 18–20.

Watkins, B., Cheston, R., Jones, K. and Gilliard, J. (2006) 'Coming out with Alzheimer's disease changes in insight during a psychotherapy group for people with dementia.' *Aging and Mental Health 10*, 1–11.

Yale, R. (1995) *Developing Support Groups for Individuals with Early Stage Alzheimer's Disease: Planning Implementation and Evaluation*. Baltimore, MA: Health Professions' Press.

Yalom, I.D. (1970) *The Theory and Practice of Group Psychotherapy*. New York, NY: Basic Books.

Further reading and related references

Cheston, R. (1996) 'Stories and metaphors: talking about the past in a psychotherapy group for people with dementia.' *Ageing and Society 16*, 579–602.

Cheston, R. (2004) 'Top-dogs and Under-dogs: Marginalising Problematic Voices.' In A. Innes, C. Archibald and C. Murphy (eds) *Dementia: An Inclusive Future? Marginalised Groups and Marginalised Areas of Dementia Research*. London: Jessica Kingsley Publishers.

Cheston, R. (2005) 'Shame and avoidance: issues of remembering and forgetting with people with dementia.' *Context: The Magazine for Family Therapy and Systemic Practice 77*, 19–22.

Cheston, R. and Bender, M. (1999) *Understanding Dementia: The Man with the Worried Eyes*. London: Jessica Kingsley Publishers.

Cheston, R., Jones, K. and Gilliard, J. (2004) 'Falling into a hole: narrative and emotional change in a psychotherapy group for people with dementia.' *Dementia: The International Journal of Social Research and Policy 3*, 95–103.

Cheston, R., Jones, K. and Gilliard, J. (2006) 'Psychotherapeutic Groups for People with Dementia: the Dementia Voice Group Psychotherapy Project.' In B.M.L. Miesen and G.M.M. Jones (eds) *Care-giving in Dementia: Research and Applications 4*. New York, NY: Brunner-Routledge.

Goudie, F. (2002a) 'Trauma and Dementia.' In G. Stokes and F. Goudie (eds) *The Essential Dementia Care Handbook*. Bicester: Speechmark.

Goudie, F. (2002b) 'Working with Psychological Distress.' In G. Stokes and F. Goudie (eds) *The Essential Dementia Care Handbook*. Bicester: Speechmark.

Sabat, S.C. (2002) 'Epistemological issues in the study of insight in people with Alzheimer's disease.' *Dementia: The International Journal of Social Research and Policy 1*, 279–293.

Sutton, L. (2003) 'When late life brings a diagnosis of Alzheimer's disease and early life brought trauma. A cognitive-analytic understanding of loss of mind.' *Clinical Psychology and Psychotherapy 10*, 156–164.

Chapter 10

Art Therapy
Getting in Touch with Inner Self and Outside World

Steffi Urbas

Overview

Art therapy has been used as one component of a 'self-maintenance' rehabilitation programme for people with early stage dementia in Germany for some time (Romero and Wenz 2001). It reflects a person-centred intervention that focuses on the positive attributes of the person engaging with it. Art therapy is based on the underlying assumption that everyone can be creative at some level. The self-portraits of William Utermohlen, who has Alzheimer's disease, have raised awareness in the medical world of creativity and the brain (Crutch, Isaacs and Rossor 2001). Art therapy, however, represents a psychosocial intervention that is concerned with how people with dementia may actually benefit from art. It is suggested that art therapy allows people with dementia the time to focus, express themselves, and recapture a sense of control – all aspects of their former lives that they may have progressively lost to their disease. This chapter summarises the wide-ranging scope of art and art therapy in dementia care, and outlines how art therapy was used as an individualised psychosocial intervention at the Alzheimer Therapy Centre in Germany. The case studies describe how people with dementia have learned to express themselves through art. The examples have been selected to demonstrate some of the recurring themes that are often present in the art work created by people with dementia.

Rationale: art therapy and dementia

Art therapy can be conceptually grouped with the creative therapies that include the use of metaphor (Killick 2005), poetry, dance, song and music. These are often collectively described as the 'arts therapies' and can be used to facilitate change or 'access the person' who has reduced or absent verbal expression due to chronic neurological diseases (Waller 2002a). This chapter will specifically focus on art, to the exclusion of other forms of creative therapies, since art therapy was one of the components of an individualised self-maintenance therapeutic rehabilitative programme at the Alzheimer's Therapy Centre in Germany (Romero and Wenz 2001). It has also been evaluated in one small controlled trial of group therapy in early stage dementia in the UK (Sheppard *et al.* 1998; Waller 1999, 2001, 2002b).

Art has emerged as an important therapeutic activity that can provide a channel of communication (MacGregor 2005) and in the UK there are a number of Alzheimer's Society projects where volunteers and people living with dementia and family carers use art to enjoy relationships (Driver 2005; Mitchell 2006; Neal 1996). These dementia care art projects occur in a variety of settings such as drop-in centres (Mitchell 2006), within ordinary community facilities (Driver 2005), as one-off voluntary sector ventures (Baker 2004), at day units using paid staff and therapists (Benham 2004; Meadows 2004; Ridley and Parker 1996; Wilson 2001) and within hospitals (Tyler 2002). Some projects include family carers as volunteers or participants (Driver 2005; Mitchell 2006; Neal 1996).

The types of art used to support people with early dementia range from pleasurable activity within art classes (Driver 2005), modelling at a heritage centre (Mitchell 2006), making murals over a week at an Alzheimer's Society premises (Neal 1996), making collages and creative rugs as an activity at a day hospital (Meadows 2004), developing an individualised banner with the help of an artist and occupational therapist at a day hospital (Baker 2004), using a self-expression closed group at a day hospital to express the experience of dementia (Benham 2004) and, with the help of trained art therapists, to express the painful emotions that are encountered in the course of dementia (Osler 1988; Waller 1999).

Art therapy has been used with young and older people who have dementia (Cossio 2002; Falk 2002; Tyler 2002; Waller 1999, 2002b) and can be applied within groups (Cossio 2002; Falk 2002; Tyler 2002; Waller 1999, 2002b) or within individual sessions (Liebmann 2002; Tyler 2002; Wilson 2001).

The next section describes art therapy as an early individualised psychosocial intervention, which contributes to the self-maintenance rehabilitation programme at the Alzheimer Therapy Centre in Germany.

Getting in touch with inner self and outside world

Art therapy is a form of non-verbal psychotherapy that uses visual imagery where the processes of painting, drawing or sculpting provide a space for individual expression and creative engagement with the self in action and social engagement. It is therefore concerned not just with experiencing a fulfilling encounter with the self, but also with satisfaction of a basic human need for active and successful engagement with the environment. These two cornerstones of quality of life are, in general, rarely experienced by people with Alzheimer's in their everyday life. It is the art therapist's task to offer a therapeutic space providing experiences that address these basic needs. This is achieved through sensitive understanding of individual resources and needs, strengths and preferences.

The pictures that accompany this chapter were initially prepared as large colour paintings. Each originally formed part of a series of pictures demonstrating the encounter with the self and with the outside world that can take place in the context of art therapy. They have been chosen because, even when presented as small monochrome images as they are here, they still convey powerful emotions. Even though they cannot explain the developing process of therapy, they still provide an insight into the varied possibilities of the therapeutic work.

Without words

In art therapy it is possible to express ideas and feelings that cannot be conveyed in words. This is particularly important in the case of people with language impairments. Art therapy works with the striving and protestation of the spirit as it seeks expression and audience. Listen to the lament of a clergyman experiencing the early signs of Alzheimer's disease:

> Sunken in lonely darkness
> In the hidden hours
> I am silent towards heaven
> And stay dumb.
>
> My words fail me
> My memory is vanishing

I am lost in a
Ghetto of silence.

I can no longer express myself
In the darkness of memory of speechlessness
I seek my memory and speech.

Yet one thing remains –
My soul protests
About accepting the bitterness,
A broken, already spiritless life.

The theme of being shut off from contact with the environment, trapped in an individual world of increasing speechlessness, is pervasive for people with Alzheimer's. This is expressed in the picture titled 'Without Words' (Figure. 10.1), painted by a man with early stage dementia. He had allowed himself to be ensnared by the verbal limitations imposed on him as a result of the illness, and had begun to react with depressive withdrawal and sarcasm towards himself and towards life in general. As his art therapist, at each session in the studio, I presented him anew with the challenge of facing the unexpected vicissitudes of life. From simple painting on A4 pages to the joint development of a big group picture, from watercolours and brush to finger painting with the

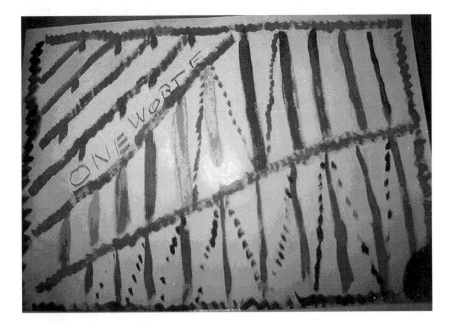

Figure 10.1 'Without Words'

whole hand, to making a mask for a fancy-dress event, he dared over and over again to overcome his own shadow. In an informal setting that offered care and respect, this intellectually oriented man overcame his 'But I can't do that!' and 'But that's silly!' and increasingly discovered pleasure in spontaneous expression. The repeated expression of a creative impulse, which he very consciously accepted as psychologically beneficial, seemed to kindle in him a new sense of courage, and a belief that he could triumph over obstacles. At the end of therapy he spoke of a flame, which he experienced as something new in himself, and which he wanted to keep alive through engaging in a range of activities.

Dancing around one's inner being

Art therapy can help people with dementia to make contact with their inner being, enabling them to find and develop their own inner resources. During free painting with no specific instructions, irrespective of the stage of illness, circular shapes frequently emerge. In producing these circular shapes, one person moves the brush with a sweep, another quite cautiously, the next with a flourish, another with intense concentration. The mandala always rotates around a central point – clarity and simplicity in a life that is characterised by confusion as familiar associations disintegrate. Often the mandalas grow from the inside out with each new revolution, just like the opening of a flower. The experience of painting is an expansion of the self which creates space – a therapeutic progression – especially for people who feel small and frightened because of the nature of their illness.

Angela, a shy and timid woman, sketched her first pictures very fast, almost as if she was frightened to take too much time for herself. But soon she was dancing during the development of her mandalas (Figure 10.2) with a happy smile on her face, and taking more and more time for herself.

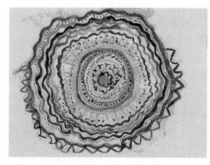 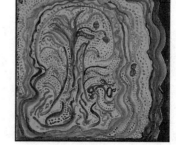

Figure 10.2 Angela's 'mandalas'

Strengthening the self through repetition

People with dementia are known to be masters of repetition. Often they can feel trapped in their repetition. Even more frequently, they feel hurt when their carers react with an abrupt 'Not that again!' Listen to the words of one man as he 'recovered' from his knowledge of having a progressive dementia:

> When a few islands emerge amidst a fog of fleeting memories, perhaps at any given moment just a single island onto which I can jump, then that's what I do. By continually seeking it out and telling myself and others about it, because I can remember it, even if I don't know anything about it, I enable this memory to stay alive. Naturally I want to be sure of my island, my anchor in a sea of forgetting!

The image above allows the therapist (and even the family carer) to go along with the person with dementia in their tendency towards repetition. By going along with the person, not just patiently but enthusiastically, using the repeated construction of a motif, the therapist can enhance a sense of security in the person with dementia. After a stay at the Alzheimer Therapy Centre, for example, one man with advanced dementia continued, with considerable perseverance and with the greatest of pleasure, to draw a whole series of pictures that were composed 'only' of straight, horizontal lines.

Repetition of a motif can often show us, in quite a dramatic way, what the central elements are in the way a person experiences his or her world. Often it is possible to discern a personal theme which the person needs to communicate to the outside world and to make real to him- or herself. A priest, for example, painted a church in almost every picture, and sometimes two. In so doing, he expressed the steadfastness of his faith. He came right to the point when he said, 'I am a religious man, after all.' The same man went through a phase in which he repeatedly expressed a vivid memory of a holiday through different variations on a particular motif (Figures 10.3).

Acting on spontaneous impulses and instincts

'Free painting' is a central component of my art therapeutic work with people who have dementia. This involves me giving them as much space as possible, and the minimum possible amount of instruction and help. It also means that on the whole (not least because of obvious signs of apraxia or an expectation of apraxic difficulties), I encourage people to engage in abstract expression. People with dementia who in their daily lives receive regular feedback on all the things they are doing wrong, are encouraged, while painting, to follow their own immediate impulses and to trust their own instincts. Where this is

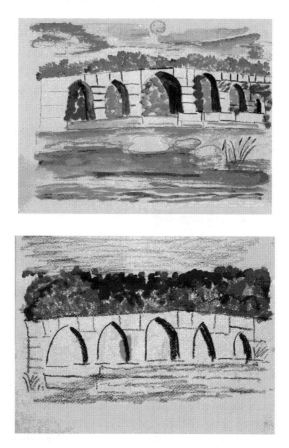

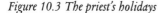

Figure 10.3 The priest's holidays

successful, the encounter with oneself can be deep and therapeutic. The end result is a set of paintings which, by aligning with the individual's life force, represents authentic self-expression and communicates the painter's individual strengths.

Betty had mild dementia with good verbal abilities but noticeable apraxic difficulties. It was she who went to the doctor because she had noticed changes in herself, and it was she who insisted that the doctors take her seriously. She appeared to be a very determined woman, and she argued a great deal with her husband, who was caring for her. She described herself as 'a fighter', and on the one hand she was proud of this, but on the other she also acknowledged that she often made life difficult for herself and others. In therapy, she worked on this theme very independently, with striking results. In contrast to her expectations ('That's definitely not for me!') she quickly took pleasure in 'free painting' and gained confidence in her artistic abilities. Then, one day, she came to therapy with a determined expression on her face, intending to paint a beautiful picture of sunflowers. Unhappy with the first attempt, she tried hard at a second, with similar results. In discussion afterwards she said, 'I got an idea into my head again, and I thought I absolutely had to make it come out – typical!' and seemed relieved. At this point she made a conscious decision to treat herself more gently, and from then on she painted with eager spontaneity and joyful discovery. In doing so, she restricted herself to one colour at any one time. 'Otherwise I'll just get wound up about which colours go together,' she explained. Each time she was newly astounded at her efforts. Full of pleasure, she would talk about the emerging evidence of her motivation along the following lines: 'I had nothing definite in mind. The pictures just emerged from inside me.'

Expressing and presenting self

Artistic activity produces therapeutic results where the individual's present life force is facilitated and developed, reaching expression in a picture, a model, or perhaps simply in a gesture. It is about the experience of facing up to oneself, getting to know oneself, and accepting oneself. Moreover, the experience of achieving expression through creative activity is a means of presenting the self to others. When they are able to enter into this process observantly, therapists can experience something of and through the person who has brought the creative work into being. Art therapy creates ways of getting in contact with the inner self and with the outside world.

Conclusion

The examples described outline common themes that are observed when using art therapy with individuals who have dementia, that is, expression of oneself without words, making contact with the inner self to facilitate change, strengthening the self through repetition, acting on spontaneous impulses and instincts and expressing and presenting the self. Through artistic endeavours, people with dementia can reacquaint themselves with spontaneous 'let yourself go' enjoyment. This is important on a number of levels. It allows the person to 'scratch beneath the surface' of their disease and dig deeper to remind themselves of their capabilities, and get to know themselves again. They have the opportunity to do something for fun, which demands only that they 'have a go', and which allows them to be as creative and imaginative as they wish. On another level, however, as they focus and engage with the task at hand they can regain a sense of control, belief in themselves, and perhaps courage. In addition, their art work can act as self-expression, at a time when this may not be available to them through any other means.

Acknowledgements

Art therapy as used at the Alzheimer's Therapy Centre described in this chapter is based on a talk given at the Alzheimer Europe 10th Anniversary Meeting, Munich, October 2000, and is an adapted translation of the German-language text published in the *Proceedings of the Alzheimer Europe 10th Anniversary Meeting.* The chapter has been updated by the editors since its inception in 2001.

References

Baker, S. (2004) 'How the arts can reveal a stairway of hope: Sandwell Third Age Arts.' *Journal of Dementia Care 12*, 6, 21.

Benham, L. (2004) 'How the arts can reveal a stairway of hope: an abstract.' *Journal of Dementia Care 12*, 6, 20.

Cossio, A. (2002) 'Art Therapy in the Treatment of Chronic Invalidating Conditions: From Parkinson's Disease to Alzheimer's.' In D. Waller (ed.) *Art Therapies and Progressive Illness.* Hove: Brunner-Routledge.

Crutch, S.J., Isaacs, R. and Rossor, M.N. (2001) 'Some workmen can blame their tools: artistic change in an individual with Alzheimer's disease.' *The Lancet 357*, 2129–2133.

Driver, B. (2005) 'Art in action.' *Journal of Dementia Care 13*, 6, 21.

Falk, B. (2002) 'A Narrowed Sense of Space: An Art Therapy Group with Young Alzheimer's Sufferers.' In D. Waller (ed.) *Art Therapies and Progressive Illness.* Hove: Brunner-Routledge.

Killick, J. (2005) 'Making sense of dementia through metaphor.' *Journal of Dementia Care 13*, 1, 22–23.

Liebmann, M. (2002) 'Working with elderly Asian clients.' *Inscape 7*, 2, 72–80.

MacGregor, K. (2005) 'Activities that paint a thousand words.' *Journal of Dementia Care 13*, 6, 19–20.

Meadows, G. (2004) 'How the arts can reveal a stairway of hope: art and craft.' *Journal of Dementia Care 12*, 6, 21.

Mitchell, R. (2006) 'Meet Angus and Theresa.' *Journal of Dementia Care 14*, 2, 5.

Neal, D. (1996) 'All things bright and beautiful.' *Journal of Dementia Care 4*, 1, 21.

Osler, I. (1988) 'Creativity's influence on a case of dementia.' *Inscape*, Summer, 20–22.

Ridley, C. and Parker, J. (1996) 'A promise of things to come: the Grange Day Unit mural project.' *Journal of Dementia Care 4*, 1, 22–24.

Romero, B. and Wenz, M. (2001) 'Self-maintenance Therapy in Alzheimer's Disease.' In L. Clare and R.T. Woods (eds) *Neuropsychological Rehabilitation in Dementia.* Hove: Psychology Press.

Sheppard, L., Rusted, J., Waller, D. and McInally, F. (1998) 'Evaluating art therapy for older people with dementia: a control group trial.' *Group Analysis 39*, 517–536.

Tyler, J. (2002) 'Art Therapy with Older Adults Clinically Diagnosed as Having Alzheimer's Disease and Dementia.' In D. Waller (ed.) *Art Therapies and Progressive Illness.* Hove: Brunner-Routledge.

Waller, D. (1999) 'Art therapy: a channel to express sadness and loss.' *Journal of Dementia Care 7*, 3, 16–17.

Waller, D. (2001) 'Art therapy and dementia: an update on work in progress.' *Inscape 6*, 2, 67–68.

Waller, D. (ed.) (2002a) *Art Therapies and Progressive Illness.* Hove: Brunner-Routledge.

Waller, D. (2002b) 'Evaluating the Use of Art Therapy for Older People with Dementia: A Control Group Study.' In D. Waller (ed.) *Art Therapies and Progressive Illness.* Hove: Brunner-Routledge.

Wilson, P. (2001) 'Going with the flow: art workshops for everyone.' *Journal of Dementia Care 9*, 4, 14–15.

Further reading and related references

Beaujon-Couch, J. (1997) 'Behind the veil: mandala drawings by dementia patients.' *Journal of the American Art Therapy Association 14*, 187–193.

Kamar, O. (1997) 'Light and death: art therapy with a patient with Alzheimer's disease.' *American Journal of Art Therapy 35*, 120–121.

Khan-Denis, K. (1997) 'Art therapy with geriatric dementia clients.' *Journal of the American Art Therapy Association 14*, 194–199.

Steritt, P.F. and Pokorny, M.E. (1994) 'Art actvities for patients with Alzheimer's and related disorders.' *Geriatric Nursing 15*, 155–159.

Tingley, N. (2002) 'Art as Therapy for Parkinson's.' In D. Waller (ed.) *Art Therapies and Progressive Illness*. Hove: Brunner-Routledge.

Urbas, S. (2000) 'Kunsttherapie mit Demenzkranken.' In Deutsche Alzheimer Gesellschaft (ed.) *Forttschritte und Defizite im Problemfeld Demenz*. Referate auf dem 2. Kongreß der Deutschen Alzheimer Gesellschaft, Berlin, 9–11 September 1999. Berlin: Deutsche Alzheimer Gesellschaft.

Chapter 11

A Host of Golden Memories
Individual and Couples Group Reminiscence

Irene Carr, Karen Jarvis
and Esme Moniz-Cook

Overview

The evidence base for the effectiveness of reminiscence in dementia care is thin, since not many robust studies have been carried out (Woods *et al.* 2005). However, reminiscence as both a group activity and a method of interacting with people with dementia and their families remains popular, as seen in the pan-European 'Remembering Yesterday, Caring Today' reminiscence project which was evaluated by Bruce and Gibson (1999a). Practical suggestions for working with people with dementia, including training materials, have been developed (see, for example, Disch 1988; Gibson 1994a, 1994b; Murphy 1994, 1995; Norris 1986) and Age Exchange, based in London, has been particularly active in this area (Bruce, Hodgson and Schweitzer 1999; Schweitzer 1993, 1998, 1999). The therapeutic purposes of reminiscence and the need for adequate training and supervision when carrying out this type of work have also been emphasised (Bender, Bauckham and Norris 1999) and family carers are increasingly becoming involved in reminiscence therapy (Woods *et al.* 2005). In this chapter we describe individualised, in-home, family-based reminiscence and a couples group programme for older people with early dementia and their families. Two case studies are presented using in-home life story work and collage as methods of maintaining family relationships, pleasure and identity in early dementia. The couples group programme, 'Rekindling the Past – Enlivening the Present' facilitated by two Alzheimer's Society volunteers, with people and their families from the Hull Memory Clinic and its evaluation, are then described. This couples group programme developed by the volunteers was used as an early intervention to enhance new pleasurable activity and social relationships for both the person with dementia and their primary family carer.

Pan-European studies of the use of reminiscence for people with dementia living at home (see Schweitzer 1999) and in care homes (see Penhale *et al.* 1998) have been supported by the European Commission, with projects involving local communities, volunteers and the arts. Activities such as individual or group reminiscence, oral history, life review and life story work all share some commonalties which may be included within the broad umbrella of reminiscence (see Bornat 1994). Whilst definitions can be somewhat blurred, reminiscence has been broadly seen as follows:

> Groups of older people…whose main concern is the retrieval of past experiences and its recording and preservation in some way can be said to be taking part in oral history. When those same groups share memories with a view to understanding each other, or a shared situation, or with the aim of bringing about some change in their current lives, they are involved in reminiscence work. (Murphy 1994, p.1)

Given this definition, it is hardly surprising that reminiscence has usually been carried out as a group activity. Life review, life story work and collage, on the other hand, tend to be undertaken as one-to-one or triangulated activities, involving the individual together with perhaps a close family member or friend and a facilitator or co-ordinator of the activity. Whilst, as we shall see later, there is a place for group-based reminiscence as an early intervention, individualised family-based reminiscence can have an important place in reinforcing family relationships. In the early stages of a dementia the relationship between the person and their primary family supporter (e.g. a spouse or adult-child), can become subtly undermined due to word-finding problems, reduced conversation and social withdrawal, all of which are seen by the family as 'changes in the person'.

When the diagnosis of dementia is provided, for example, in the context of a memory clinic, it is important that people are supported to maintain normal interpersonal routines and lifestyles, whilst actively using adaptive coping strategies such as 'the fighting spirit' and 'dementia disease minimisation' where necessary, in order to maintain self-confidence, esteem and a sense of self. Individualised family-based reminiscence activities, such as life story work, may therefore be more suitable than an organised group activity, for use with people and their family or friends, in the earlier stages of dementia.

As the term 'life review' implies, an integral part of this activity is the review and evaluation of past life events and the use of past experiences to help cope with some of life's transitions and the milestones of old age. Life story work (Murphy 1995; Murphy and Moyes 1997) is an equally individualised approach, but with perhaps a wider scope of potential rehabilitative benefit and opportunity. To some extent it can be viewed within the discipline of health promotion, since health is defined as 'a resource for living rather than merely the absence of disease' (World Health Organisation 1986). It can be used proactively to develop and maintain relationships, to promote conversations and pleasurable activity and to enhance psychological well-being. As the disease progresses it can provide a visual resource to help the person with dementia and others to maintain a sense of the person's identity and enhance communication and relationships. Life story work can take a number of forms including the production of tangible end points such as reminiscence boxes, life story books and collages.

Life story books and collage not only dwell on personal narrative but also employ a rich source of sensory cues to encourage positive expression in individuals who can thus tell their own unique life stories. This may include both factual and anecdotal reflections on their past and present lives and possible hopes and aspirations for the future. In this way the project can become a pleasurable, positive and meaningful activity. Elizabeth Shipway describes how, when she was clearing out her mother's flat following the move into residential care, she began a life story book with her mother. During the shared activity, her mother was able to forget her distress at having to leave her own flat, and eight months later they had reached 1936 in the 'journey' of their shared book (Shipway 1999). Murphy (1995) suggests that the product of life story work, whether this is a book or collage or whether it takes some other format, should never be put aside as completed, as to do so would be to imply that the individual's life is over, or without hope.

Collage work, pioneered in the city of Hull, UK, like life story books, has its theoretical roots within the reminiscence literature in general and life review in particular (see Bruce *et al.* 1999). It may, however, also be associated with the developing range of creative approaches to dementia care, such as the therapeutic use of the arts (Killick and Allen 1999; Lawrence 1998; Neal 1996; Waller 1999; see Chapter 10 of this volume), which may be a way of promoting self-expression as a form of communication and as an activity of aesthetic intent (Allen and Killick 2000). In Hull, collage has been used as a therapeutic activity with older individuals with and without dementia in a clinical mental health setting (see, for example, Jarvis 1997, 1998a, 1998b; 2000a, 2000b), with staff in enhancing personal relationships with people with challenging behaviour in dementia (Moniz-Cook, Woods and Richards

2001) and also as one aspect of group activity described later in this chapter, within the 'Rekindling the Past – Enlivening the Present' couples group project. The procedure itself differs from other types of art and collage work in dementia care, such as group collage (see, for example, Bruce *et al.* 1999, p.42; Jagger 2000), making group murals (Neal 1996) and art therapy group work (Waller 1999). As with life story books, collage also aims to enhance the self or identity of the person with dementia, and there are many similarities between this way of working and using a life story book. However, the end product is different, since it is displayed on one large sheet or poster (see Jarvis 2001 and Figure 11.1), rather than in the format of a book or folder. It may be more suitable for people whose fear has precipitated mood and associated cognitive problems with attention. Assessment for the best method of life story work (i.e. books, collages or boxes) should be considered in the context of the person's circumstances (Murphy and Moyes 1997) as we shall see in the two case studies presented. The use of life story books and collage as an early intervention with people with dementia within their family context will be considered next.

Developing life story books and collage

Developing life story books and collage can be used as a pleasurable therapeutic process, to stimulate conversation, to reinforce and demonstrate retained skills, to validate and reinforce personal achievements and also as a cathartic prompt. Once developed, life story books are equally effective as a personal expression of oneself, a memory aid, a conversation tool for use with family and friends, a means of providing distraction and/or reassurance during episodes of distress and even as a record of the individual's life for future generations.

The simplest form of a life story book or collage reflects a collection of anecdotes, pictures and personal memorabilia. These artefacts can have particular symbolic meaning for the person. For example, one person included a small square of flannelette, which reminded her of her days as a young mother when she tucked her daughter up at night. Another individual's life story book contained a strongly smelling polishing cloth which he had used regularly to clean his car during his long years as a driver. It is not always necessary to focus overly on the written narrative, since for some people, particularly those with dysphasia, this may reduce their interest and ownership of the activity. Equally, any narrative that is used in a life story book should, as closely as possible, represent the individual's usual terminology and language, since a worker's personal interpretation may lead to the need for the individual to overly focus on the dialogue, thus reducing spontaneity and potentially limiting its future use as a memory prompt. For similar reasons it is not always important to rely too heavily on factual accuracy when developing life story books or collage. An overview or 'snapshot' of a meaningful recollection or event is often far more productive.

Although essentially a fluid and flexible process, a number of key stages are usually observed in conducting life story book or collage work. For example, it is essential to establish the person's, and if appropriate, the carer's, willingness and motivation to carry out the activity. Often this can best be achieved by careful explanation and practical demonstration of other consenting individuals' life story books or collages. Once consent has been established, the visual format, title and general presentation of the book should be discussed with the individual and, if they so wish, with the family or friend. This is followed by mutually agreeing the topics, taking care to actively avoid past regrets and upset for both the person and the family member. Often the discussion follows the person's life milestones, such as schooldays, family life, holidays, and so on, prior to perhaps the most enjoyable part of the activity: talking, reflecting, exploring ideas and gathering the memorabilia which may be used to create the book or collage. However, when developing a life story book or collage it is not necessary to go through all of the person's life stages and it is more important to draw out the one or two aspects of life that have particular pleasure and meaning for the person. These are often related to family, work or certain hobbies. Once the decision has been made to create a life story it is important that the therapist provides structure to enhance the use of resources, but does not direct or lead the person, since this is the person's or couple's own expression of identity and relationships or picture.

Life story books and collage
Should these be used with everyone who has dementia?

It is not suggested here that life story books and collage, or indeed reminiscence itself, are appropriate for everyone. Indeed, it is important to consider through a careful evaluation of the person and family who may not benefit, or indeed who may become unduly distressed by the process of life review and reminiscence (Bender *et al.* 1999), before deciding to develop a life story book or collage. Sensitivity to potential contraindications of the use of reminiscence in dementia, before discussing the possibility of either of these procedures, is important. This may be achieved by allowing time for a relationship to develop between the therapist and the person and his or her family.

Collage and life story books are clearly not always possible with people who have serious visual impairment. Furthermore, certain topics that may arise during the making of a life story book or collage, as with reminiscence and life review in general, may cause distress in people with dementia who have experienced past trauma. In people with dementia who may have frontal lobe damage, there is then the risk that the person might perseverate on (i.e. get stuck on the theme of) the past trauma which may then be difficult to resolve, resulting in exacerbated distress for the person. It is also important to consider past and previous family tensions and relationships prior to beginning life story work. For example, one person required reassurance throughout that her ex-husband would not be able to access her life story book.

The choice of format, content, impetus and how it is used are all important considerations prior to engaging in life story work (Murphy and Moyes 1997). If an adequate psychosocial assessment has occurred, we suggest that there is a growing window of opportunity to achieve greater effectiveness with people in the earlier stages of dementia for whom, despite difficulties in retaining new memories, old memories and some aspects of conversation often remain relatively accessible.

Similarly, collage has been used with people with and without dementia. One example of its use is with a terminally ill person, where it provided a meaningful way of addressing life issues for the person and became a treasured keepsake for the relative (Jarvis 1997). Benefits include reduction in anxiety and depression, and improvements in self-esteem. Descriptions of life story collage and its positive outcomes with individuals with dementia and their families can be found in Bruce *et al.* (1999, p.28) and Jarvis (1998a, 1998b; 2000a, 2000b).

Next, two case vignettes are presented to demonstrate the use of life story books and collage. The first describes a person who was referred to the Hull Memory Clinic for early diagnosis and possible intervention. A life story book complemented other equally important psychosocial interventions during quite a traumatic and demanding period of his life. The second describes the use of collage with a person who was referred to a community mental health team for older people, and was supported by a community psychiatric nurse and staff at a day hospital for people with dementia. Here, his collage helped him to interact with his son when the effects of dementia and anxiety had disrupted their relationship.

Out of the shadows
Eric and Mary and their family's life story book

Eric, a stoic 70-year-old man, was referred by his GP to the Hull Memory Clinic in October 1997 as a result of his wife's growing concerns about his absent-mindedness and reduced initiative. Meeting the couple for assessment was in itself both interesting and enjoyable for the staff. Mary was a gregarious extrovert, flamboyantly dressed and keen to take centre stage. Eric, the person who was referred, on the other hand, was strong and silent, with a dry sense of humour. It quickly became apparent that he had been his wife's 'rock' throughout their life together and had protected and generally supported her through any number of 'madcap' (their terminology) ideas and schemes.

This loving couple had an only daughter, married with one son (known affectionately as his grandmother's heartbeat!). Not surprisingly, given the energy and drive that the couple portrayed, their daughter saw them as somewhat larger than life figures and could not easily comprehend their potential decline or ultimate mortality.

Eric's diagnosis of vascular dementia of approximately three years' duration, therefore, came as an enormous shock to them. His wife desperately wanted to continue their happy life together and to find ways for Eric to avoid making simple yet annoying mistakes, like leaving the front door open and not putting the milk back in the fridge. His daughter needed much more emotional support and education about prognosis and coping. She was open to new ideas and responded well to advice and demonstration provided by the memory clinic nurse. Thus she understood the need to avoid 'deskilling' her father, and the importance of helping him to manage life using well-rehearsed routines and external memory aids to prevent or compensate for common errors. These strategies were extremely successful in managing practical aspects of his daily life. However, they were powerless to address the family's emotional loss of their 'rock and mainstay', whose personality and character they began to describe as 'shadowy' and less defined. Nor did these interventions enable Eric to explain and express his own insight into his difficulties and fears for the future.

It was therefore suggested to him that he might like, with support from his family and the memory clinic nurse, to develop a life story book, which would be a special piece of work that he, as the biographer, would take the lead in. He was keen to take up this challenge and spent many happy hours in lofts, garages and cupboards finding photographs and memorabilia.

The ensuing discussions proved to be an animated and humorous inclusion to his usual routines. He and his wife were able to laugh together at each other's past failings and triumphs. Conversation became easier between the couple and the family began once again to see Eric's underlying character, his retained skills and ultimately his need for emotional support.

Some weeks into this process Mary became increasingly unwell and was subsequently diagnosed as having a secondary brain tumour. Following two major operations she died, some six months later. Throughout her deterioration the life story book was regularly brought out, reminisced over and added to. It also served as an emotional cue and cathartic prompt shortly following Mary's death. Despite being totally bereft, Eric was unable to find either the right words or responses to his own grief or that of others. His sister-in-law, in particular, found this distressing and could not, therefore, easily communicate or offer her support. However, with encouragement, he described and talked to her about his married life with her sister, and a new companionable level of grief and understanding was reached, which helped a little in the overall process of grieving and moving on. With support from family, community services, regular routines, and memory prompts, Eric has successfully managed day-to-day activities and still, surprisingly, remains in his own home. Unfortunately, his physical health has recently deteriorated (as is often the case in vascular dementia where co-morbid physical health problems can be prominent) and he may require permanent residential care in the next year or so. One can only speculate at this stage whether his personal life story book might be supportive in ensuring a smooth transition on to the next stage of his life, when that occurs. It is hoped that either ourselves and/or his daughter may help him to use his book to enable care staff to understand him as a person and to assist him in the adjustment to the social environment of the care home.

From anger to laughter
Harold and his son's improved communication using collage

Harold had been suffering with memory loss for over a year. His son was the main carer, living at home and looking after both his father, Harold, and his mother, who had very poor physical health.

Harold attended a day hospital and also had periodic respite care, although he did not enjoy being away from home. When at home, Harold spent his time repeating himself, often argued and sometimes lost his temper. He was in denial about his memory problems and whilst this minimisation of his problems may have served him well (see Stokes 2000, p.57); it appeared to place a strain on his son's ability to cope.

When the community psychiatric nurse visited Harold at home, it quickly became clear how much he enjoyed reminiscing. Together with the nurse, Harold looked at photographs that were special to him and talked about his memories. Harold provided her with photographs and other memorabilia that he had selected. She obtained photocopies, and from these she assembled his collage. When Harold was shown the collage, he was clearly moved; his eyes filled and he immediately spoke about everything on it with fondness. On a later visit he stated that it was so precious to him that he was going to include it in his will, with a clear indication of who should inherit it.

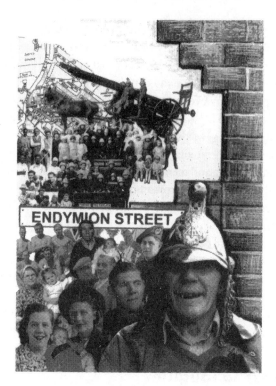

Figure 11.1 Harold's collage

Harold's son reported that their relationship had improved. He said that when Harold became fixed on an idea, or began arguing, the collage provided an easy way of changing the content of their conversation from negative to positive. Harold's short-term memory problems did not affect his ability to talk about the collage, or his recall of events surrounding the collage content. Any conversation about the collage clearly lifted his mood and following this Harold was frequently observed to be laughing or joking with others. Clearly his presentation had changed, which in turn reduced the burden and stress experienced by his son.

Validating past experience and present personhood

Whatever the format of the end product (a book or a collage), life story work allows individuals with memory difficulties or early stage dementia to 'tell' their own unique stories and to reflect on their past and future lives. It is important to remember, however, that these are mere tools, and attention needs to be paid to the way in which they are used (Murphy and Moyes 1997). Engaging with people with dementia and their families using therapeutic life story work and reminiscence will continue to require sensitivity as well as training and supervision (see Bender *et al.* 1999; Bornat 1994).

In the case studies described above, different formats (i.e. a book and collage) were used for people with early dementia who had different psychosocial circumstances, and the impetus to do the work came from within a relationship between the nurse and the person with dementia. In both cases the content was guided by the person, and in the first case the changing circumstances within the family allowed the work to remain ongoing and to help with adjustment to a life transition. In both case studies the life story book and collage contributed to the provision of positive interaction and emotional experiences. Life story work allows validation of both past experience and present personhood, and the person's sense of 'self' may be strengthened through these creative and enjoyable activities. Use of these creative methods of self-expression may have an important role in counteracting the disease model of dementia that is often associated with the diagnostic process undertaken in the early stages of a developing dementia. This process may, for some people with dementia, result in withdrawal and social isolation and ultimately depression, particularly if the relationship between the person and the family is undermined as families progress to becoming 'carers'. Life story work in the early stages of dementia provides the context for pleasurable but powerful activities that may help to prevent the extra disabilities that are often a consequence of reduced self-confidence and social withdrawal in people, and acceleration to becoming a 'carer' for the family member.

Couples group reminiscence: 'Rekindling the Past – Enlivening the Present'

Providing emotional support for people with early dementia through group therapy is an important early intervention (see Jones, Cheston and Gillard 2002), but it is also helpful for some people and their families to also meet with others, in order to reinforce normal social relationships through engaging in pleasurable activity. Structured reminiscence is a shared activity that most people can engage in, including those who have poor conversation skills, as there are always aspects of the past that can provide pleasure. It therefore lends itself to early group-based psychosocial intervention, for those people and family members who have become socially isolated due to the subtle interpersonal and social consequences that can arise from the insidious changes in early dementia.

The 'Rekindling the Past – Enlivening the Present' group reminiscence programme for people who were diagnosed at the Hull Memory Clinic with an early dementia, and their family (or friend) was developed at the Hull Drop-in Memory Centre in 2002, by two volunteers from the local Alzheimer's Society. The primary objective of the couples group programme was to promote pleasurable social activity and interpersonal communication through structured reminiscence, with the family carer acting as 'therapist' and both the person and the carer contributing to the natural social context that is required to promote new relationships and thus reduce social isolation. The centre's objectives were to provide an enriched psychosocial venue with activities that could maximise the positive resources of people with dementia and their families. Thus, where a person and their primary family supporter or carer had indicated at the point of diagnosis that they had (a) lost pleasure in each other due to the developing dementia or (b) become fearful of being apart from each other, or (c) become socially isolated, bringing them together within a reminiscence group with others was seen as a way of providing an enriched pleasurable social environment for both the person and the family.

People below the age of 65 and their spouses who fitted this profile were initially included. However, all of these declined to continue after the first session. They reported that reminiscence activities did not bring them pleasure, but instead exacerbated their fear of ageing and dementia.

In order to establish the groups, the following prerequisites were needed:

- access to community transport

- a regular meeting place with a telephone point of contact between sessions for families to raise questions and concerns

- a comfortable, suitably furnished room

- availability of space including another quiet room to talk privately at breaks

- a large table for collage and group work

- television and video availability for themed discussions

- easy access to refreshments and toilets.

Three groups were conducted by two facilitators including one who was a former family carer, over a period of 12 months. Up to five couples participated in each group and in each case people were matched to groups based on their personal customs, culture, everyday life interests and age. Most participants used their own transport, taxis or community transport, and each session took place on an afternoon from 1.30 pm to 3.30 pm. The weekly sessions were devised to follow largely biographical experiences with sessions two to eight acting as a time for participants to select meaningful material that they would use for their end product, i.e. the life story book and/or the collage. The ten-week session plan is shown below, but for each group this was adjusted to follow participants' customs, interests and past experiences:

- *Week 1*   Introductions/Getting to know you

- *Week 2*   Schooldays

- *Week 3*   Work

- *Week 4*   Marriage/Family/Celebrations

- *Week 5*   Happy holidays/Days out/Memories of favourite films and shows

- *Week 6/7*   Visits to significant places in Hull such as the docks, significant streets or participant's demonstration of favoured activity (baking, embroidery or shipping collection exhibitions); hobbies

- *Week 7/6*   Visiting speaker with a one-twelfth scale model of a 1950s terraced house and an 'open all hours' shop, used to promote discussion and for some groups to arrange visits

- *Week 8*   Memories of the war (this was not included in all groups but incorporated within sessions two to five, allowing an extra session to cover content of week six)

- *Week 9*   Commence collage/life story book

- *Week 10*   Complete collage/life story book.

Keeping activities inclusive and relevant were core principles of the groups. As facilitators got to know the participants and learned of their life experiences, relevant memorabilia were sourced to encourage participation and memories. Well-planned activities to stimulate discussion are an important stimulus (Bruce and Gibson 1999b) and theme-based activity was included in each session. Session five was particularly well received as it engaged a local charity which made creative miniatures of past local shops and homes. This allowed participants to recall their past dwellings, which some subsequently visited and photographed for their collage. Following a teabreak, a facilitated discussion covered what particular memorabilia were important to each couple and might be included in their life story. The session ended with written homework and a summary of arrangements for the following week.

A case study of couples group reminiscence

One group consisted of four men with an early dementia and their spouses. The men were keen to do something to improve their memory but also wished to please their wives, who they were aware had taken on more day-to-day activities since they had developed memory problems (see Chapter 12 of this volume). Their wives, on the other hand, were keen that their partners had 'social stimulation' as according to them the spouse was 'no longer himself' and had withdrawn from conversation and social activity. They were also themselves somewhat lonely, as they were sad about their perceived loss of companionship, since their husband 'was no longer the man they knew'.

Group attendance allowed the subtle but negative effects of dementia on family carers to become balanced by the joint celebration of good times past and the realisation that it was possible for a person to change but also to retain valued aspects of their identity. For example, one previously reserved man enjoyed telling the group about his time at the docks and his animation surprised and gave much pleasure to his wife who had not heard him talk freely for many months. There were also numerous examples, especially during weeks three to five, and the final sessions, when couples demonstrated their sense of commitment and gratitude towards each other (Schweitzer 1998).

To assist the men in understanding the relationship between memory and reminiscence they completed a pre-group measure using the Autobiographical Memory Interview (AMI, Kopelman, Wilson and Baddeley 1990), followed by attendance at a talk on autobiographical memory as compared to other forms of memory, prior to the couples reminiscence group. The AMI measures a person's recall of facts from their own past life (Personal Semantic Schedule, PSS) and recall of specific incidents (Autobiographical Incident Schedule, AIS). Table 11.1 shows the Autobiographical Memory Interview results for each of the four men prior to and following group-based reminiscence.

Table 11.1 Results of Autobiographical Memory Interview (AMI) scores				
Name	Pre-intervention score		Post-intervention score	
	PSS	ASI	PSS	ASI
Len	32	3	30	1
George	48	24	57	27
Eric	50	11	50.5	16
William	57.5	13	61	14
Total	187.5	51	198.5	58

The total group scores on the AMI improved post intervention, and for three men both the PSS and AIS scores improved. George's ability to recall actual facts from his past life improved quite significantly, much to his pleasure. Not only was detail more accurate, but the information was also recalled more frequently. Eric's ability to recall facts remained largely the same, but the richness of his recall for autobiographical incidents was enhanced and his pleasure as he described events was evident.

The men themselves enjoyed meeting each other and they and their wives continued to maintain their friendships, with the other group members and group members wives' respectively, after the group ended. Two couples began a regular outing to the swimming pool and two others joined a walking club together. All four couples met at each other's homes for tea approximately once a month in the year that followed. Additionally, two couples scanned their collage and had these framed for family members, whilst one made Christmas cards for family with theirs.

Practical guidelines for developing life story books and collages

Full guidelines for making a collage may be found in Jarvis (2001). The advice that follows should be considered in the making of either a life story book or a collage:

- Decide on the format – life story book or collage – based on a careful psychosocial assessment and discussion with the person.

- Think in advance about potential family tensions or obstacles that might hinder the person in developing and using their life story work.

- Avoid unhappy or disturbing events, sadness or loss, including past trauma and situations of failed relationships. Reassure the person that you are only interested in aspects of their past that they wish to share with the people they choose.

- For life story books, spend some time with the person agreeing what the book should be called and how it should be presented. For example, Gladys wanted to call her book 'My Book of Memories', whilst Jane called her book ' My Life Story'. In terms of presentation, Gladys used a green ring binder with a picture of a rose (her favourite flower and the name of her sister) on the cover. Jane used a painting that she had done in the past for the cover of a scrapbook which reflected her chosen theme of past achievements as a mother and homemaker who enjoyed baking, floral arrangements and painting watercolours.

- Ensure that the person is allowed the time to select the photographs and any other materials they might want to include. If there is repetition in the material, or there are copious amounts of materials, discuss whether one or more collages would be appropriate. There could be different themes incorporated in one large collage, or several collages representing different themes that are important to the person. Similarly, different pages or sections in a life story book could represent different themes.

- If there is a general theme, additional source material can be found in newspapers or magazines. For instance, if the person loves gardening, seed packets and pictures of plants or pressed flowers could be used, but it is always important to discuss the selection process with the person and, if appropriate, with the family.

- For life story books, it is important to use large text and to use the person's own style and vocabulary in written material.

- With the person's permission, photocopy or scan original photographs and materials in order that the originals may be returned to the person or family. Colours can be varied or tints can be used; sepia colour themes can be discussed if the person has any preferences. The focus should be on the person's colour preferences and not the staff's. Colour itself has significance in different religions. Some people may be superstitious and may attach meaning to certain colours, or the person may be reminded of something by a particular colour (see Stokes 2000, pp.104–105 with regard to purple; Moniz-Cook *et al.* 2001, the case of Jack and the colour green).

- Encourage the person to participate as much as possible – with collage, by laying out the materials to form a picture for the collage, and for a life story book by participating in decisions on presentation, in laying things out and in sticking in photographs. Think about and negotiate sizes and colour schemes to best convey the theme or the individual's preferences. For the collage, agree on the final arrangement before adhesion – a spray type of adhesive is a user-friendly medium, though other glues can be used and may be more cost effective.

- The finished collage and the cover of a life story book can be laminated. This is practical as it does not tear and can be wiped clean. Some people have enjoyed framing their collage as a permanent memento for the future.

When beginning collage work and life story books, the following items of equipment are likely to be useful:

- Choice of potential coloured ring binder folders, scrapbooks and specimens of specially designed photograph albums that are often available from bookshops. The latter may be somewhat restrictive but can be useful for some people who have particular preferences. Examples of these are:

  o Short, P. (1993) *My Life Story*. Springfield Leisure Art Collection, 47 Yarborough Road, Wroxall, Isle of Wight, PO38 3EA.

  o Short, P. (1993) *Memory Diary*. Springfield Leisure Art Collection (address above).

  o Pettigren, J. and Woodin, M. (1992) *From Grandmother with Love*. London: Little Brown.

  o Pedersen, J. and Taylor-Smith, A. (1995) *Grandparents' Book*. London: Four Seasons.

  o Sheppard, L. and Rusted, J. (1999) *A Pocket Book of Memories*. London: Hawker Publications.

- Coloured pencils or pens.

- Paints.

- Scissors or scalpel.

- Glue stick or adhesive spray.

- Coloured paper or card (A3 is a good working size and practical for photocopying) for collages.

- Self-healing mat, or thick pad for cutting materials on.

- Metal ruler.

- Paper to laminate.

- Scanner and colour printer.

Conclusion

Developing an identity-reinforcing product through life story books and collage can be a means of enhancing pleasurable in-home family relationships and reducing interpersonal anxiety or social withdrawal in early dementia. However, engaging people in new group activity including reminiscence can be problematic, as many people with early dementia are fearful of 'showing themselves up' (Moniz-Cook and Vernooij-Dassen 2006). Structured couples group reminiscence set in acceptable social and physical environments has the potential to counteract this fear and also provide the social context for new relationships, particularly where people and their families have become socially isolated. We suggest that structuring reminiscence as a group activity to include shared events from the past, including those that bring pleasure, is the intervention of choice if introducing people with dementia and families to new social situations and groups is the identified goal for rehabilitation. The functions of home-based and couples group reminiscence may differ in early dementia, but the enjoyment and therapeutic benefits of enhanced social confidence and reduced carer distress remain an important means of preventing excess disabilities in dementia. Our experience in the Hull Memory Clinic early intervention programme suggests that the reminiscence activities we used were not appreciated by younger people with dementia and their families.

Acknowledgements

Thanks to Joan Rennardson and Christine Elston (Alzheimer's Society, Hull Branch), who developed and conducted the couples group reminiscence programme between 2002 and 2005 at the Hull Drop-in Memory Centre.

The 'Rekindling the Past – Enlivening the Present' couples reminiscence project was pioneered by Joan Rennardson, who was successful in obtaining an After Dementia: Millennium Award Grant to run the project.

References

Allen, K. and Killick J. (2000) 'Undiminished possibility: the arts in dementia care.' *Journal of Dementia Care 8*, 3, 16–18.

Bender, M., Bauckham, P. and Norris, A. (1999) *The Therapeutic Purposes of Reminiscence.* London: Sage.

Bornat, J. (ed.) (1994) *Reminiscence Reviewed.* Maidenhead: Open University Press.

Bruce, E. and Gibson, F. (1999a) 'Remembering yesterday: having fun, making friends.' *Journal of Dementia Care 7*, 3, 28–29.

Bruce, E. and Gibson, F. (1999b) 'Remembering yesterday: stimulating communication.' *Journal of Dementia Care 7*, 2, 18–19.

Bruce, E., Hodgson, S. and Schweitzer, P. (1999) *Reminiscing with People with Dementia: A Handbook for Carers.* London: Age Exchange.

Disch, R. (ed.) (1988) *Twenty Years of the Life Review: Theoretical and Practical Considerations.* New York, NY: Howarth Press.

Gibson, F. (1994a) *Reminiscence and Recall.* London: Age Concern Books.

Gibson, F. (1994b) 'Reading around…reminiscence.' *Journal of Dementia Care 2*, 3, 24–25.
Jagger, B. (2000) 'Roses all year in memory lane.' *Journal of Dementia Care 8*, 5, 16.
Jarvis, K. (1997) 'I remember me.' *Signpost 2*, 3, 18–19.
Jarvis, K. (1998a) 'Recovering a lost sense of identity.' *Journal of Dementia Care 6*, 3, 7–8.
Jarvis, K. (1998b) 'The way we were.' *Nursing Times 94*, 38–39.
Jarvis, K. (2000a) 'Collage and memory.' *Community Practitioner 73*, 5, 593–594.
Jarvis, K. (2000b) 'Stolen moments.' *Nursing Standard 14*, 16–17.
Jarvis, K. (2001) *Collage and Dementia: A Practical Guide for Carers and Care-workers.* London: Alzheimer's Society.
Jones, K., Cheston, R. and Gilliard, J. (2002) 'Sharing problems through group psychotherapy.' *Journal of Dementia Care 10*, 3, 22–23.
Killick, J. and Allen, K. (1999) 'The arts in dementia care: tapping a rich resource.' *Journal of Dementia Care 7*, 4, 35–38.
Kopelman, M., Wilson, B.A. and Baddeley, A. (1990) *Autobiographical Memory Interview.* London: Harcourt Assessment.
Lawrence, L. (1998) 'Using the arts to cross boundaries.' *Journal of Dementia Care 6*, 2, 22–24.
Moniz-Cook, E., Woods, R. and Richards, K. (2001) 'Functional analysis of challenging behaviour: the role of superstition.' *International Journal of Geriatric Psychiatry 16*, 45–56.
Moniz-Cook, E. and Vernooij-Dassen, M. (2006) Editorial: 'Timely psychosocial intervention in dementia: a primary care perspective.' *Dementia 5*, 307–315.
Murphy, C. (1994) *It Started with a Sea-Shell: Life Story Work and People with Dementia.* Stirling: Dementia Services Development Centre.
Murphy, C. (1995) 'This is your life.' *Journal of Dementia Care 3*, 2, 9–10.
Murphy, C. and Moyes, M. (1997) 'Life Story Work.' In M. Marshall (ed.) *State of the Art in Dementia Care.* London: Centre for Policy on Ageing.
Neal, D. (1996) 'All things bright and beautiful.' *Journal of Dementia Care 4*, 1, 21–24.
Norris, A. (1986) *Reminiscence with Elderly People.* Bicester: Winslow Press.
Penhale, B., Bradley, G., Parker, J., Manthorpe, J., *et al.* (1998) *EQUAL: Enhancing the Quality of Life of People with Alzheimer's Disease. Final report for the European Commission under the Action for Alzheimer's Disease Framework.* Hull: University of Hull.
Schweitzer, P. (1993) *The Reminiscence Handbook: Ideas for Creative Activities with Older People.* London: Age Exchange.
Schweitzer, P. (1998) *Reminiscence in Dementia Care.* London: Age Exchange.
Schweitzer, P. (1999) 'Remembering yesterday: a European perspective.' *Journal of Dementia Care 7*, 1, 18–21.
Shipway, E. (1999) 'Creating a life story book.' *Alzheimer's Disease Society Newsletter*, February, 4.
Stokes, G. (2000) *Challenging Behaviour in Dementia. A Person-Centred Approach.* Bicester: Winslow Press.
Waller, D. (1999) 'Art therapy: a channel to express sadness and loss.' *Journal of Dementia Care 7*, 3, 16–19.
Woods, B., Spector, A., Jones, C., Orrell, M. and Davies, S. (2005) 'Reminiscence therapy for dementia.' *The Cochrane Database of Systematic Reviews*, Issue 2. Chichester: Wiley.
World Health Organisation (1986) *Ottawa Charter for Health Promotion.* Ottawa, ON: Canadian Public Health Association.

Further reading and related references

Keady, J., Clarke, C.L. and Adams, T. (eds) (2003) *Community Mental Health Nursing and Dementia Care: Practice Perspectives.* Maidenhead: Open University Press.
Marshall, M. (ed.) (1997) *State of the Art in Dementia Care.* London: Centre for Policy on Ageing.
Schweitzer, P. (2005) 'Making memories matter: a project of the European Reminiscence Network.' *Dementia 4*, 450.
Thorgrimsen, L., Schweitzer, P. and Orrell, M. (2003) 'Evaluating reminiscence in dementia care.' *Journal of Dementia Care 11*, 5, 35–36.

Chapter 12

Developing Group Support for Men with Mild Cognitive Difficulties and Early Dementia

Jill Manthorpe and Esme Moniz-Cook

Overview

Within an early detection and intervention service for people aged over 65 years with memory impairments in the north of England, practitioners became aware of a number of men who had few opportunities to meet other men in this position. Most had an early dementia and all were living in their own homes. These men were at risk of developing depression, due to social withdrawal because of their perceived cognitive difficulties. This had resulted in a reduced social life and undermining of their social identities. The opportunity to meet men in a similar position of their own generation, in their own homes on a regular basis, was thought likely to increase social activity, reduce social isolation and, in the longer term, reduce the risk of depression. This chapter describes the setting up and organisation of such groups, the content and experiences during meetings and the outcomes for members.

Rationale: background and evidence for a men's group

People with dementia living at home when compared with those without dementia, tend to have reduced social networks, increased family contact and less time spent with friends, neighbours and community groups (Wenger

1994). This is not surprising as there is a 'routine and unremarkable compo-nent of family life' (Forbat 2005, p.18) that family members should take care of each other. While men are increasingly more likely to be carers, because they are now living longer than in the previous decade, normative gendered expec-tations about the role of women in caring still exist.

There is a wealth of literature on the beneficial effect of experiential social support and, more recently, self-help groups (Chapter 9; Henderson 1990; Lees 2006; Mills and Bartlett 2006). Groups can provide support, contact with others, stimulate people to think, feel and act, and meet the psychological and social needs that we all have (Bender, Norris and Bauckham 1987; de Klerk-Rubin 1995; Mason, Clare and Pistrang 2005). They may develop into opportunities for service users to offer service providers feedback and advice in health and social care provision. They can also provide an informal opportu-nity for people to discuss their problems if they wish. Socially oriented groups and activities have the potential to engage people who are in the early stages of a disability or illness to adjust to loss of skills and confidence.

In many parts of the UK, contact or support groups for people with dementia exist in most localities and knowing how to get in touch with them for support is perceived to be one of the advantages of early diagnosis (Iliffe and Manthorpe 2004). While the existence of stigma surrounding the label of dementia may contribute to reluctance in thinking about discussing dementia outside the family, support groups are more prevalent than individual counsel-ling for people with early stage dementia in the UK, although, as Cheston (1998) observed, this may be as much a matter of resource efficiency as the proven efficacy of a given type of group. Whilst group opportunity is growing, it is still the case that they are only available to a minority (Mason *et al.* 2005).

It is known that individuals differ in their experiences of receiving a diag-nosis of dementia and that these take place in the context of relationships. However, apart from a few accounts (see Pearce, Clare and Pistrang 2002; Rainsford and Waring 2005; van Dijkhurzen, Clare and Pearce 2006) there is surprisingly little discussion of the impact of gender in groups. More women than men have dementia, and women are often majority users of services and compose the bulk of practitioners in health and social care. Professions such as social work, for example, largely consist of women working with women (White 2006). Older women seem to find using services more acceptable than men (Scott and Wenger 1995) and this may be because they are used to being in female environments. Local contexts are also likely to be important in demo-graphic profiles of service users. For example, in areas where early male mor-tality is high, notably in poorer and former industrialised localities in countries such as the UK, men may not be major users of services for people in later life.

Dementia care service users and practitioners, for example, often contain much greater proportions of women than men. Commentators therefore argue that this helps to account for inadequate prioritisation and resources within services (Bender 2003). This context may affect service uptake by perceived minority groups, such as men. In addition, widowed, divorced and never married men, for example, often have more restricted social networks, engage in more health risky behaviours, and are more materially disadvantaged than older married men (Age Concern Surrey 2006). All these characteristics may mean that they are not likely to join groups of their own volition. In supporting their sense of identity, men may prefer different forms of social involvement as compared with women (Davidson, Daly and Archer 2003). They also appear to delay in their access of health professionals (Davidson *et al.* 2003). Thus, gender continues to structure male experiences and activities. Furthermore, work on the experiences of being widowed in later life has found that some men find it hard to recover their lost contacts with friends and that their support networks may decrease in size as they age (Chambers 2005; Davidson 2000).

Some services have developed activities that acknowledge diversity among their user groups. These include groups or activities for carers, for younger people with dementia, for people from particular ethnic groups or cultures. With the 'discovery' (Fisher 1994) of male carers, social and health care services in the UK began to see gender as an important social-demographic characteristic among older people. The Age Concern Surrey report (2006, p.40), for example, describes a group for older men in a social centre that has made sustained efforts to attract men, by having speakers and a more explicit structure in an effort to be more acceptable. Archibald (1994) reported that 'special' places for men in service settings may help them feel less constrained and may enable them to talk about shared interests or backgrounds. Not all men, of course, wish to socialise with other men and a cautionary note was made by Age Concern Surrey that sometimes practitioners over-emphasised men's desire to mix in male company:

> Professionals were inclined to stress the need for men to be able to meet other men, but many (by no means all) of the men interviewed were keen to meet with women as they missed female companionship. (Age Concern Surrey 2006, p.13)

Dementia and risks of depression

Feelings such as turmoil, helplessness, and diminished self-esteem are often evident when people with newly recognised early dementia talk together in support groups (Snyder *et al.* 1995). Receiving a diagnosis of dementia with the breaking of the bad news may contribute to depression, even when people have strong social supports. Facing the prospect of losses may emerge quickly, possibly compounded by the reactions of others, and the individual affected may ponder on their implications. The risk of depression is high. One UK study estimated that 63 per cent of people with Alzheimer's disease also have depression symptoms (Burns, Jacoby and Levy 1990). Another, from the USA, found that 30 per cent of people with Alzheimer's disease met the criteria for major depression (Teri and Reifler 1987). Bender (2003) notes the impact of the collapse of assumptions as a person begins to realise that his or her memory is failing, then starts to realise that his or her body and brain are no longer functioning properly and that everything in life feels uncertain and potentially unstable.

Clearly many of the discussions that practitioners might have with a person who has early dementia – about their future wishes, or about fulfilling some of their ambitions and dreams, or about making plans for their living arrangements and finances – may be matters that might prove difficult for a person with depression (Manthorpe and Iliffe 2005). Such a person may not feel up to attending some of the support groups that provide self-help or those with therapeutic aims. As is seen in the groups described by Cheston, Jones and Gilliard (2006; Chapter 9), many such groups provide a valuable social function. However, this very characteristic and the way the group is publicised may be worrying for some people with depression. To counteract such reluctance, while acknowledging people's rights to makes their own decisions, practitioners Manthorpe and Iliffe (2005) recommend that practitioners try the following:

- Offer to take and stay with a person during the group.

- Encourage relatives or carers to make use of support groups even if the person they are supporting does not want to attend, or attend with them (Chapter 14); set up one-to-one professional or volunteer visits at home, equipped with an outline of a support group's programme, to provide the person with the same information, to some degree, until they feel ready to attend one.

- Ask another member of the group to make contact with the person before the group, so as to reduce the worry of not knowing anyone.

- Talk to group leaders about their possible difficulties and ways of accommodating a person with depression in some or all of the group's activities.

Being in a minority in any such group may be a cause of anxiety – for example, the only man in such a setting may feel very isolated or self-conscious. The voluntary sector in England has recently observed that its activities are often perceived as 'feminised' and that there is a lack of front-line male staff or volunteers (Ruxton 2006).

Developing men's social groups

Keady and Nolan (1995) noted that approaches to dementia care are increasingly focusing on carers' needs. They argued for a focus on the person with dementia, especially in the early stages. The groups described in this chapter were attempts to provide a structure whereby men could develop coping strategies to manage their memory loss and associated disability. While relief or a break for their family carers was an added spin-off for some, the aim of person-centred groups can be to offer support to men with early dementia in a context where they may feel some affinity with their peers. For current generations of men, a common experience of national service or enlistment may be unifying to a degree and most men have also several decades of work or trade experiences (see Box 12.1).

Box 12.1 Background of three men in one group

Thomas: Used to be a carpenter. He talked about an isolated occasion of 'getting lost' for seven hours. The police and his friends were out looking for him. He said he was not lost but he had wanted to go for a long walk and had walked to his previous home. He said he enjoys going for a walk each day. He walks about 10 to 12 miles a week.

William: Used to be an accountant. He retired about ten years ago and is now 80 years old. He has two children, a son and a daughter. He was in the armed services for nearly ten years, where he met his wife in Italy.

Alan: Left school at the age of 14 years. He then worked in a cinema selling confectionery. He did this for about two years and was then promoted to work as a projectionist. Alan continued with this job until he was called up to go into the Air Force. When he left the service he decided he did not want to work nights again and turned his hand to working for an electronics company. Alan stated that he did many jobs within this company and remained with them until his retirement.

The introductory chapter of this book notes that groups for people with dementia may have a number of functions. These may include provision of psycho-educational or social support, cognitive stimulation, psychotherapy, and reminiscence.

The aims of the pilot men's social group outlined by Sainsbury, Gibson and Moniz-Cook (1996) and considered here were devised by staff at a memory clinic consisting of a memory nurse and a psychologist. Plans were made to achieve the following aims:

- to increase socialisation and prevent or reduce withdrawal

- to provide an opportunity to meet peers with similar difficulties, in non-threatening environments, thereby normalising their difficulties and providing support

- to maintain memory by increasing activities

- to promote fun and enjoyment

- to 'normalise' carer relief or breaks and their perceptions about dementia at an early stage (thus reducing fatalism and the therapeutic nihilism that can predominate in dementia care management).

The pilot group

Men may be invited to join such groups because of their similarities in being at an early stage of the dementia trajectory. In the pilot group described here, four men were in the early stages of a dementia and another man had mild cognitive impairments and functional difficulties which resulted in similar problems of social withdrawal. The memory team decided to run the group in the members' own homes, with agreement from the men and their wives, to ease any anxiety and normalise the activity. The group initially met once a week for eight weeks. After this it was envisaged that they would continue for a further three weeks, with the dementia team staff providing transport. Following this, it was hoped that the group would become self-supporting, making use of transport provided by volunteers.

The structure of the meetings was decided by the group during the first sessions (facilitated by the staff) and a list of ideas for activities was generated. At the end of each meeting, the group decided where they would meet next week and what they wanted to talk about or do. This led to suggestions of outings to a local army transport museum and to ten-pin bowling.

Each session was summarised at the end and information was provided about the next meeting. This was sent in the form of a personalised letter to each member after each meeting, to aid memory and to maintain interest. Duff and Peach (1994) evaluated mutual support groups for people who were in the early stages of a dementia, and their participant feedback also highlighted the fact that written invitations and reminders were useful practical strategies.

Evaluation of the pilot group

Before the first meeting, each man was asked to complete the Happiness, Confidence and Affect self-rating scales questionnaire (adapted from Burns 1989). In addition, they were asked to complete a Social Situation self-rating questionnaire, to examine feelings about recent social encounters. For all of these measures, positive scores are reflected by higher ratings on the scale. Measures were repeated at meeting four and again at meeting eight, the last of the formal meetings. After each session, the facilitators rated each person on the scale below:

- *Attentiveness* – the degree to which participants appeared interested in the group.

- *Responsiveness* – the degree to which participants responded to stimulus material, discussion or prompting.

- *Spontaneity* – the degree to which participants offered contributions of their own.

- *Involvement* – the degree of non-verbal response to group activity.

- *Interaction* – the degree of interaction with other members of the group.

- *Anxiety* – the degree of anxiety before and during the group meeting.

A composite score for each person was then calculated.

Outcomes

Attendance was high, although one man missed four of the later sessions due to ill health. Throughout the group meetings, a steady improvement in the men's involvement, general socialisation and ability to concentrate and cope with this social situation were noted. The men remembered when the group was taking place, the names of other participants and what they wanted to do or talk about. This was particularly encouraging, given that four of the men had an early dementia. Gerber *et al.* (1991) also reported similar findings.

However, improvement in this setting was not reflected to the same extent in the men's self-reports of how they felt about other social situations. The four men who remained in the group reported only slight improvements in their feelings about social encounters. This could be due to changes in their expectations of themselves, insensitivity in the questionnaire, or the short length of time between ratings.

Self-ratings of their happiness and confidence showed no change, apart from one person who reported increased happiness as the sessions progressed. Mike Bender (personal communication) commented that six to eight weeks in a group would not be long enough to show a change in confidence. The self-reported affect scale showed a variety of results, with one person reporting a decrease and another reporting an increase. However, all scores remained high. There was one decrease on the affect scale. Given that deterioration might be expected in some of these scales, it may be that the group helped to prevent deterioration, but the period of time was very short.

The group seemed to provide a 'normalising' experience for many difficulties that the men were experiencing, and insights into the everyday problems these can cause. The extent to which this happened was encouraging, given that this was not the primary aim of the group.

Lessons from the pilot

Looking back, the staff identified several aspects of the group that they felt needed to change in any similar development. For instance, the men were initially uneasy with the informal nature of the group. Groups may benefit from a more structured format at the beginning, gradually changing to an informal structure as members become more familiar with each other. This has been seen in examples where planned time-limited psycho-educational groups have developed into long-term social support groups (Bender 2006). Furthermore, comments from one group member, a few weeks into the group, revealed that he remained isolated by his impression that he was the only person with memory difficulties, since no one had talked about their memory problems. The group structure could facilitate discussion of how particular memory difficulties affect each person, with the aim of increasing awareness of their similarities. As the group shifted to independence, a man who was more outgoing than the others said he felt pressured to keep the conversation going within the group. With the benefit of hindsight, it would have been helpful to have had another person with a similar personality in the group to assist with this, if possible.

At the end of the group, the facilitators were able to gradually withdraw and arrangements were made for the group to be self-supporting. The staff felt that continuing the group would be particularly important, in the light of research which suggests that improvements may not be maintained once a group has ended (Gerber *et al.* 1991). Other groups may benefit from repeating evaluations to examine the group process, through interviews with the group members after the facilitators withdraw. This could enable insight into whether groups and any of the improvements noted continue and what factors may promote this. The capacity and willingness of the voluntary sector in taking on transport and other organisational tasks also need to be considered further and it should be included in planning such developments and service design from the start.

Groups where participants are more closely matched for personality and history might be possible. Evaluation could include measures of self-efficacy, general anxiety and depression (to see if there is a beneficial effect on mood) and perhaps focus more directly on the effects of group processes, on enhancing feelings of control and adaptive coping in early dementia. Choices about evaluating dementia care are often limited by resources and have to consider a range of communication and ethical issues (Murphy 2007), but they can nonetheless be empowering for participants and practitioners alike. Feminist research methods are generally more familiar in social and health care research settings. Evaluation of men's services will need to consider the gender of the facilitators as well as the researchers, and the ways in which men are able to design or influence studies that draw on men's perspectives.

Four more men's groups have since been held. The latest group (held in 2007) put into practice changes based on some of the lessons learned. For example, early attention was given to what the men would want from the group sessions (see Box 12.2 for examples of their views). One theme that has emerged from the five groups carried out so far is the importance of wives' practical and emotional support (see Box 12.3). This has led us to think that while the group may be termed a 'men's group', it is a group of married men, and thought would need to be given to how to involve men who are not living with a female partner or who are not in heterosexual relationships (Manthorpe and Price 2003).

Later groups have not been held in members' own homes. This is because of emergency transport difficulties and the problems these locations posed for the families of group members over time. When men were not able to attend or their families to 'host' the group, this resulted in lack of continuity and problems with organisational rearrangements. The current resolution is that the men's groups are held in community centres, pubs, or a drop-in service. Access to public transport and parking is essential.

Box 12.2 What would you like from these group sessions?

William: To converse with people in the same situation.

Alan: When talking to others that don't have memory problems it is different to talking to people that are in the same boat as you (have memory problems).

Thomas: We are all in the same boat, same problems.

Alan: You don't realise that there are people out there with the same problems. You are not on your own.

Box 12.3 The importance of wives

Thomas: Our wives have really good memories. We all find it helpful to be able to talk about our problems and how people get round it.

William: There is an army of us with memory problems.

Alan: If you try to hide your memory problems, it makes your memory worse. I leave notes for myself if I want to remember things; I write it on a piece of paper and put it in my pocket. When you forget something, the harder you try to remember it the worse your memory gets.

William: When you start worrying about it, it has a greater effect on you.

Thomas: I do not worry about memory, my wife is always on standby for me.

Alan: I think we would all be lost without our wives, we do not realise how much we rely on them. If my wife goes out I worry about what happens if the phone rings. How will I remember the message? Usually it is okay because I know the people and I know the answers to the questions.

All: We have not been talking about anything specific but we have been just talking. This is keeping our brains active.

The role of the facilitator has continued to be important but, when asked, the men have so far not expressed a wish specifically for a male or female facilitator. This proves easier in arranging staff attendance. Continuity of facilitator is also helpful, but less important if the venue is a service setting, since the 'sense of stability' provided by availability of other staff has been identified as important for support groups (Mason *et al.* 2005).

The final lesson from the early groups is that a men's group will only continue if there is active support from and for their wives. They need to be reassured that the group is safe, that they will not be excluded from the service, and that support will be available in the long-term.

Conclusion

We are beginning to be more aware of the importance of the social context in which awareness of dementia is experienced and expressed (Clare *et al.* 2006, p.142). Gender mediates such experiences, and support groups for men may be services that are commissioned at local level. If this is so, thought will need to be given about the staffing of such services and ways in which men who do not want to participate are not excluded from other generic services. The experience of the pilot and other groups is that there are benefits, but that such groups are resource intensive. We suggest that more thought needs to be given to how men are welcomed into early dementia services and the images that such services convey in terms of their publicity and illustrative activities. In this way men may be more likely to see that their minority status may not be reasons for self-exclusion and will be empowered to address behaviours, expectations and activities that are not meeting their needs.

Acknowledgements

We thank psychologists Louise Sainsbury, Gillian Gibson, Hannah Wilkinson, Jas Harrison and Marcus Tredinnick at the Hull Memory Clinic for reporting on their work as group facilitators and allowing us to make use of their insights and experiences. We thank the people using the clinic's services for their willingness to contribute to this study.

References

Age Concern Surrey (2006) *Investigation into the Social and Emotional Wellbeing of Lone Older Men.* Guildford: Age Concern Surrey.

Archibald, C. (1994) 'The trouble with men…' *Journal of Dementia Care 2,* 1, 20–22.

Bender, M. (2003) *Explorations in Dementia: Theoretical and Research Studies into the Experience of Remediable and Ensuring Cognitive Losses.* London: Jessica Kingsley Publishers.

Bender, M. (2006) 'The Wadebridge Memory Bank Group and beyond.' *PSIGE – Psychology Specialists Promoting Psychological Wellbeing in Late Life – Newsletter 95,* 28–33.

Bender, M., Norris, A. and Bauckham, P. (1987) *Groupwork with the Elderly: Principles and Practice.* Nottingham: Nottingham Rehab Limited.

Burns, A., Jacoby, R. and Levy, R. (1990) 'Psychiatric phenomena in Alzheimer's disease, III: disorders of mood.' *British Journal of Psychiatry 157,* 81–86.

Burns, M.C. (1989) 'Correlates of psychological well-being among caregivers of dementing and non-dementing elderly relatives.' MSc dissertation, University of Leeds.

Chambers, P. (2005) *Older Widows and the Lifecourse: Multiple Narratives of Hidden Lives.* Abingdon: Ashgate.

Cheston, R. (1998) 'Psychotherapeutic work with people with dementia: a review of the literature.' *British Journal of Medical Psychology 71*, 211–231.

Cheston, R., Jones, K. and Gilliard, J. (2006) 'Psychotherapeutic Groups for People with Dementia: The Dementia Voice Psychotherapeutic Project.' In B.M.L. Miesen and G.M.M. Jones (eds) *Care-giving in Dementia: Research and Applications,* Vol. 4. London: Routledge.

Clare, L., Markova, L., Romero, B., Verhey, F., *et al.* (2006) 'Awareness and People with Early-stage Dementia in 2006.' In B.M.L. Miesen and G.M.M. Jones (eds) *Care-giving in Dementia: Research and Applications,* Vol. 4. London: Routledge.

Davidson, K. (2000) 'What we want: older widows and widowers speak for themselves.' *Practice 12,* 1, 45–54.

Davidson, K., Daly, T. and Archer, S. (2003) 'Older men, social integration and organisational activities.' *Social Policy and Society 2,* 2, 81–89.

de Klerk-Rubin, V. (1995) 'A safe and friendly place to share feelings.' *Journal of Dementia Care 3,* 3, 22–24.

Duff, G. and Peach, E. (1994) *Mutual Support Groups: A Response to the Early and Often Forgotten Stage of Dementia.* Stirling: University of Stirling, Dementia Services Development Centre.

Fisher, M. (1994) 'Man-made care: community care and older male carers.' *British Journal of Social Work 24,* 659–680.

Forbat, L. (2005) *Talking about Care: Two Sides to the Story.* Bristol: The Policy Press.

Gerber, G.J., Prince, P.N., Snider, H.G., Atchinson, K. *et al.* (1991) 'Group activity and cognitive impairment among patients with Alzheimer's disease.' *Hospital and Community Psychiatry 42,* 843–845.

Henderson, A.S. (1990) 'The social psychiatry of later life.' *British Journal of Psychiatry 156,* 645–653.

Iliffe, S. and Manthorpe, J. (2004) 'The recognition of and response to dementia in primary care: lessons for professional development.' *Learning in Health and Social Care 3,* 5–16.

Keady, J. and Nolan, M. (1995) 'IMMEL: assessing coping responses in the early stages of dementia.' *British Journal of Nursing 4,* 309–314.

Lees, K. (2006) 'Gentlemen who lunch: developing self-help groups for people with early diagnosis of dementia.' *PSIGE – Psychology Specialists Promoting Psychological Wellbeing in Late Life – Newsletter 96,* 33–37.

Manthorpe, J. and Iliffe, S. (2005) *Depression in Later Life.* London: Jessica Kingsley Publishers.

Manthorpe, J. and Price, E. (2003) 'Out of the shadows.' *Community Care,* 3 April, 40–41.

Mason, E., Clare, L. and Pistrang, N. (2005) 'Processes and experiences of mutual support in professionally led support groups for people with early-stage dementia.' *Dementia 4,* 87–112.

Mills, M. and Bartlett, E. (2006) 'Experiential Support Groups for People in the Early to Moderate Stages of Dementia.' In B.M.L. Miesen and G.M. M. Jones (eds) *Care-giving in Dementia: Research and Applications,* Vol. 4. London: Routledge.

Murphy, C. (2007) 'User Involvement in Evaluation.' In A. Innes and L. McCabe (eds) *Evaluation in Dementia Care.* London: Jessica Kingsley Publishers.

Pearce, A., Clare, L. and Pistrang, N. (2002) 'Managing sense of self: coping in the early stages of Alzheimer's disease.' *Dementia 1,* 173–192.

Rainsford, C. and Waring, J. (2005) 'Support groups offer a lifeline.' *Journal of Dementia Care 13,* 3, 13–14.

Ruxton, S. (2006) *Working with Older Men: A Review of Age Concern Services.* London: Age Concern England.

Sainsbury, L., Gibson, G. and Moniz-Cook, E. (1996) 'It's good to talk – man to man.' *Journal of Dementia Care 4,* 5, 20–22.

Scott, A. and Wenger, C. (1995) 'Gender and Social Support Networks in Later Life.' In S. Arber and J. Ginn (eds) *Connecting Gender and Ageing: A Sociological Approach.* Maidenhead: Open University Press.

Snyder, L., Quayhagen, M.P., Shepherd, S. and Bower, D. (1995) 'Supportive seminar groups: an intervention for early stage dementia patients.' *The Gerontologist 35,* 691–695.

Teri, L. and Reifler, B.V. (1987) 'Depression and Dementia.' In L.L. Carstensen and B.A. Edelstein (eds) *Handbook of Clinical Gerontology.* New York, NY: Pergamon Press.

van Dijkhurzen, M. I., Clare, L. and Pearce, A. (2006) 'Striving for connection: appraisal and coping among women with early-stage dementia.' *Dementia 5,* 73–94.

Wenger, C. (1994) 'Support networks and dementia.' *International Journal of Psychiatry 9,* 181–194.

White, V. (2006) *The State of Feminist Social Work.* London: Routledge.

Chapter 13

Group Psycho-Educational Intervention for Family Carers

Rabih Chattat, Marie V. Gianelli
and Giancarlo Savorani

Overview

A psycho-educative group intervention for informal carers of people with dementia was established in Bologna, Italy in 2000 by the Regione Emilia Romagna, and was later extended to the community-based services managed by the geriatric units of the University and of Galliera Hospitals in Genova. This chapter describes the context of this family carer group programme in Italy, the participants and programme outcomes. We conclude that, despite the reported poor efficacy for time-limited carer support groups (Knight, Lutzky and Macofsky-Urban 1993), there is a place for group-based psycho-educational interventions for family carers, if these are grounded in adequate theory and supported by empirical investigation which has used outcome measures that fit the conceptual base of the intervention programme. This study supports the Canadian randomised trial findings of Hébert *et al.* (2003), where improving carer strategies within groups appeared to minimise the potential for burden due to the development of behavioural and psychological symptoms in dementia (BPSD). The chapter concludes that early attention to carers' misunderstanding of the changes in their relatives and associated risks of isolation may be helpfully addressed by early attention to their needs at the time that the person they are supporting is in the early stages of dementia.

In Italy, as in many other parts of Europe, a high proportion of older people with dementia are cared for at home by family or unpaid carers (Murray and McDaid 2002). The stresses and strains associated with dementia care are well documented and many studies show that carers are highly satisfied with support groups (Brodaty, Green and Graham 2000), although nearly three decades of research have at best produced equivocal findings on the effectiveness of support groups for carers (Cooke *et al.* 2001; Knight *et al.* 1993; Pusey and Richards 2001). Studies that do show effects on variables other than satisfaction tend to have much more focused programmes than time-limited support groups, involving both the person with dementia and carer and with longer term flexible availability of a professional to provide support (Brodaty, Green and Koschera 2003). It is not clear whether poor efficacy is due to inadequate measurement or inadequate programmes, or both as is highlighted in an article by Lavoie (1995) entitled: 'Support Groups for Informal Carers Don't Work! Refocus the Groups or the Evaluations?'

Often support group interventions are not explicitly theory driven, results generated are apparently in conflict with one another (see Charlesworth 2001) and even in studies that have a theoretical rationale there can be an unclear relationship between theoretical frameworks and the impact of the interventions that are used. The consequence for service providers and policymakers is a difficulty in translating significant research findings into viable programmes and services at a local level (Coon, Gallagher-Thompson and Thompson, 2003a). One way of improving this situation is to focus not on improving research methodology but on how to increase the impact of intervention (Charlesworth 2001) since there have been significant improvements in efficacy of psychosocial intervention over the past 20 years (Brodaty *et al.* 2003).

Those who run support groups have little doubt that they assist family carers and the fact that people continue to attend could be taken as a marker of effectiveness. Also, the methodological evolution of research and clinical carer support groups that was highlighted by Brodaty *et al.* (2003) has begun to demonstrate movement in clinical outcomes. For example, a randomised controlled trial of a psycho-educational support group intervention involving 158 family carers showed significant effects on participant reaction to behavioural problems in their relative and the frequency of these problems also decreased (Hébert *et al.* 2003). In this study the experimental group received a theory driven cognitive behavioural group intervention lasting two hours for 15 weeks, based on the Lazarus and Folkman (1984) transactional theory of stress and coping, whilst the control group received traditional group support.

The stress–coping/adaptation theory base used in the study of Hébert *et al.* (2003) has dominated the family carer research over many years where typically measures of perceived stress and coping are used as outcomes. Other theoretical frameworks include psychodynamic approaches and a variety of social learning theories, typically including measures of self-efficacy and self-esteem as outcomes. Theory selection has been influential in deciding upon methods of intervention and the way to achieve desired outcomes and has also influenced choices of outcome measures (Schulz and Williamson 1997). However, ongoing investigations into dementia care continue to uncover the multidimensional nature of the caregiving process suggesting that either new models or building flexibility into existing ones to involve more contextually tailored outcome measures are the only way of improving our understanding of today's caregiving as a complex, dynamic process (Coon, Ory and Schulz 2003b). An example of how existing models may be developed is seen in the previously described Canadian study where the process of the intervention as well as the content was taken into account (Lévesque *et al.* 2002).

In Brescia, Italy the effectiveness of a psycho-educational group for family carers has been reported (Magni *et al.* 1995; Nobili *et al.* 2004; Zanetti *et al.* 1998a), but until recently family carer support was not a nationwide priority. In 2000, a Regional Health System Act affecting the Emilia Romagna region of Italy stated that interventions for carers were to be an essential part of the programme for developing services and intervention protocols for people with dementia. In accordance with this Act, and in collaboration with the local associations of professional and family carers of people with dementia, we developed a group psycho-educational intervention for family carers in Bologna. In this chapter we describe this intervention and present some of the outcomes achieved.

Background and rationale to programme development

Bologna, Italy where the programme was developed, was somewhat unusual for many southern European countries, including Italy, in that it comprised most of the features typical of large urban areas. There was a wide range of social backgrounds, few extended family groups, smaller sized nuclear families, a large number of dual working/income families and high divorce or separation rates, resulting in a reduction of family members who were available and willing to assist older relatives and an increasing number of non-EU citizens (usually women) acting as 'badanti' – paid care workers. Yet caregiving for people with dementia largely remained a 'family affair' (Vernooij-Dassen *et al.* 2005) mainly due to:

- the high degree of stigma attached to the condition, which still remains a barrier to using services

- low levels of recognition of the help that services can provide

- the lack of familiarity with self-help groups and group therapies in general.

The majority of family carers in Bologna conformed to the documented literature (Senesi *et al.* 1999). They were often women who were 'hidden patients' (Coon *et al.* 2003a), providing dementia care over long periods of time, reporting more physical and mental health problems, lack of sleep, additional employment complications, greater family conflict and leisure time constraints, higher use of psychotropic medications with more compromised immune systems compared to other carers or non-caregiving counterparts (see Ory *et al.* 1999; Schulz *et al.* 1995; Zarit *et al.* 1998).

Among the methods reported as most effective for translating theory into practice, we chose an approach based primarily upon knowledge and skills training. The importance of knowledge and its role as a moderator in stressful events was highlighted some decades previously by Lazarus and Folkman (1984) in their 'appraisal' concept; and by Paykel (1983) who compared the impacts of known, as opposed to unknown, events affecting coping strategies. In a psychiatric context, a 'psycho-educational' family caregiving model was proposed by Liberman (1987), who contended that caring skills and efficacy could be improved through knowledge and skills training.

We followed a model of carer distress that involves addressing primary and secondary strains, the latter referring to role change and inner conflicts, employing the three-step intervention recommended by Zarit and Edwards (1999):

1. *Information strategy,* i.e. education about dementia and its progression; impact of the disease upon individuals and their families; difficulties of caring over long periods; and resource availability.

2. *Management of stressful situations* surrounding the interpersonal relationship and emotional problems.

These two steps are thought to help carers feel more able to manage such situations and enhance their sense of control:

3. *Practical and emotional support,* which needs to be long-lasting, since this is what allows carers to feel safer over the whole course of the disease.

The programme

The educational programme was structured into ten weekly sessions of 90 minutes each. Every session addressed a main theme concerning one aspect of dementia. During the first session, led by a psychologist, the members were asked to talk about their situations and difficulties and also about their first contact with the disease, from the first symptoms up to the diagnosis and the impact of the dementia upon their well-being. The aim of this first session was to enhance socialisation and exchange of experiences not only between carers and the group leader, but also between carers themselves. During the following three meetings a geriatrician discussed some clinical aspects of dementia such as epidemiology, risk factors, types of dementia, disease course and different types of symptoms. Three more sessions, led by the psychologist, were dedicated to discussing relationships between patients and carers, difficulties related to coping, orientation and communication with their relatives, factors involved in carer distress and some of the strategies that can be used to manage symptoms, behavioural problems and stress. The remaining three sessions were led in turn by a nurse, an expert in the legal and ethical problems of dementia, and a social worker who explained the services available in the local area. At the start of each session the leader discussed the theme of the meeting for 30 minutes and the remaining time was spent by carers discussing their own questions or comments.

At the end of the course carers were offered the opportunity of taking part in a further support group. This was held monthly by a psychologist with the aim of maintaining contact, facilitating expression of emotions and supporting carers over the whole course of the disease. Sessions of individual counselling were also available at this stage, aimed at enhancing carer support and expression.

Participants and outcome

Carers were recruited in collaboration with the Association for Research and Assistance in Dementia (ARAD), the Health Agency of Bologna Nord (a local agency of the national health system) and the geriatrics unit of Galliera Hospitals in Genova. Information about the programme and invitations to carers to participate were given out through a newsletter and in a public meeting.

In Bologna the first group was run in autumn 2001, and by 2003 a further three groups with a total of 46 participants were completed. In Genova the programme was initiated in 2004 and is ongoing. The data discussed in this chapter refer to Bologna only.

The first step, i.e. the educational and training strategy, was developed with groups of 10 to 12 carers who gave their written consent to take part. All were primary carers of people affected by dementia diagnosed by geriatricians and were living in the community. Of the 46 participants, 16 were male and 30 were female. Their mean age was 57.5 years ($\pm$ 11.00, range 30 to 82 years). All had directly assisted their relatives or were involved in their care on a daily basis. Twenty-six lived with the person with dementia while 20 lived close by and were involved in daily caregiving. Thirty participants were sons or daughters while 16 were spouses. This profile may reflect the difficulty for spouses, particularly if older themselves, to participate in this type of programme, and the consequent tendency to delegate the responsibility of interacting with the external world to sons or daughters. Just over half, 54.3 per cent, had eight years schooling, and just under half, 45.7 per cent, had 13 years or more. About half of the carers were in paid employment (47%) with the remaining (53%) retired. Most were caring for female relatives (female n = 33; male n = 13), with an average age of 80.17 years (± 7.30 years, range 60 to 93 years). The average length of time that their relative had had a dementia was 4.18 years (± 2.88 years), so this was a group of relatives with a relevant experience of dementia caregiving.

Before and after the groups, participants were assessed using measures listed below, in order to tap the framework described above, i.e. the interaction between subjective factors, coping and aspects of the disease in determining stress and well-being in carers. While disease symptoms, together with socio-demographic data, can be seen as primary stress factors, coping strategies of the carer may mediate the impact.

Measures

- The Mini Mental State Examination (MMSE) for cognitive status of care recipients (Folstein, Folstein and McHugh 1975).

- The Neuropsychiatric Inventory (NPI, Cummings *et al.* 1994) is a structured interview with carers, to assess the psychological and behavioural symptoms of patients. It consists of 11 sets of neuro-psychiatric symptoms in dementia which are rated on a five-point Likert scale for frequency (how often the symptom occurs), severity (how troublesome the symptom is for the person with dementia) and the product of this, i.e. frequency multiplied by severity (the symptom level of challenge). The NPI also has a four-point Likert rating of the carers' experience of distress associated with the symptoms.

- The Caregiver Burden Inventory (CBI, Novak and Guest 1989) is a 24-item scale measured on a five-point Likert scale to assess dementia-related burden on five domains of burden in family carers. It has five subscales:

- o   physical burden: how much physical assistance is needed to support the relative and its impact on the carer's own physical health

- o   time-dependence burden: how much time is needed to support the care recipient

- o   social burden: the effect on the carer's social life

- o   emotional burden: the emotional impact experienced by the carer

- o   developmental burden: the change in their own life due to the caregiving role.

- The Coping Orientations to Problems Experienced (COPE), a 60-item, five-factor self-report scale validated for the Italian population (Carver, Scheier and Weintraub 1989; Sica et al. 1997) for coping strategies. It measures the following coping strategies: social support, problem solving, avoidance (of emotional involvement), positive attitude and religious coping.

- Socio-demographic data such as sex, age, relationship, working status, onset and duration of disease were also recorded.

Results

As seen in Table 13.1, significant improvement in carer reports of neuropsychiatric and behavioural symptoms and in coping through social support was found. Thus, carers reported lower frequency and severity of symptoms and to a lesser extent their perceptions of stress associated with behavioural symptoms were also reduced. Their emotional relief and seeking support of others also showed a significant change, probably confirming the utility of group psycho-educative interventions in satisfying some of these needs. The other domain where significant change was observed was on the problem-oriented subscale of COPE. This assesses activities and plans utilised to face problems. Here reduction in the use of problem-oriented coping was noted, suggesting that some carers became slightly over-vigilant in their search for methods to adjust to dementia. Thus it appears that the intervention offers carers more help on some aspects of coping such as social support (which also targets information-seeking behaviour) but not on others.

The most important inferences from the data indicate that a psycho-educational intervention, such as that developed in this programme, can help carers to better understand the manifestations of dementia and the different types of symptoms and can moderate reported BPSD probably through an improved ability to understand symptoms and changed attributions of their causes.

	Measure	Baseline	Post-group	P value
		Mean (sd)	Mean (sd)	
Person with dementia – cognition	MMSE	16.81 (±6.30)	17.89 (±5.57)	NS*
Carer report – frequency of behaviour symptoms	NPI Frequency	19.38 (±7.07)	14.05 (±5.65)	0.006
Carer report – severity of behavioural symptoms	NPI Severity	12.05 (±7.15)	8.15 (±4.73)	0.0004
Level of behavioural challenge	NPIF F × S	27.27 (±8.48)	17.83 (± 3.53)	0.0004
Carer appraisal/distress	NPI Stress	17.83 (±3.53)	14.50 (±3.81)	0.067
Carer – emotional burden	CBI – emotional burden	3.22 (±4.11)	2.0 (±2.16)	0.081
Carer coping using social support	COPE – social support	29.94 (±6.95)	27.76 (±6.36)	0.030
Coping using problem-solving strategies	COPE – problem-solving	32.27 (±6.28)	31.36 (±6.40)	0.051

Table 13.1 Change over time on relevant outcome measures

Note NS = Not Statistically significant

One of the most difficult problems that carers have to deal with is the sense of loss and loneliness they experience. Increased coping through social support suggests that the sessions offered carers the opportunity to meet these personal needs, through on the one hand access of information about the disease and on the other sharing their emotional burden with others in similar circumstances.

In the second part of the analysis we bring together some of the factors related to socio-demographic data and aspects of the disease associated with carer distress. The aim is to outline the role of different variables in moderating burden. Statistical analysis, application of the one-way analysis of variance (ANOVA) model, gave the following results:

1. Carers with higher educational levels were more likely to actively search for social support, use problem-solving strategies, make greater use of information-seeking strategies and accept support from others more readily. Such strategies represent more adaptive methods in coping with the situation. They reported less time dependence ($F = 2.97$; $p = 0.047$) and physical ($F = 4.54$; $p = 0.009$) burden on the CBI. Also coping strategies differ in relation to educational level, with participants with higher levels being more likely to take advantage of social support ($F = 4.84$; $p = 0.006$).

2. Carers in paid employment experienced less burden (particularly in the categories of developmental ($F = 14.85$; $p = 0$), physical ($F = 13.83$; $p = 0$) and emotional ($F = 9.96$; $p = 0.003$) burden.

3. The type of relationship between the carer and the person with dementia is important: spouses, when compared with sons or daughters, showed higher levels of developmental ($F = 10.67$; $p = 0.002$), physical ($F = 11.73$; $p = 0.001$) and emotional ($F = 11.45$; $p = 0.001$) burden.

Eighty per cent of carers who had attended the programme took part in monthly support groups and from time to time also accessed individual counselling. We have now undertaken a follow-up assessment aimed at understanding the impact of three years of educational and support programmes for carers. Although the data set is not complete, some of the inferences drawn from the follow-up interviews help in understanding the role of such interventions. When relatives were asked to express their opinions as to the usefulness of the intervention, the most frequent responses were:

1. 'It helped us to reduce the feeling of being alone with our problem.'

2. 'It helped us to be in a situation where others understand what it means to have a parent or spouse suffering from this kind of disease.'

3. 'After following the programme we can really express what is happening in our lives without fear of stigma, and we feel less need to deny or minimise.'

4. 'It offered the possibility of being constantly in contact with someone who could help us deal with our difficulties.'

5. 'It offered the possibility of developing new relationships with other people.'

An important theme that emerges from these responses is that carers express feelings of loneliness and isolation with a strong need for continuity of care and support to counterbalance the sense of abandonment by others, especially by the person with dementia himself or herself.

Conclusion

Family carer burden is less related to the stage of the dementia – particularly cognitive and functional status – than it is to carer status and the caregiving process (Montgomery and Kosloski 1999). This confirms much of current literature suggesting that the contributing factors to carer burden are less about the disease itself and more about other subjective factors, such as when the disease started, how long it has lasted, the age of carer and person with dementia, their relationship, the carer's occupational status and educational level, the quality of their prior relationship, and the potential for 'carer gain', i.e. the positive aspects of caring, all of which can moderate stress (Dunkin and Anderson-Hanley 1998; Ford *et al.* 1997; Thommesen *et al.* 2002; Zanetti *et al.* 1998b).

The frequency of behavioural and psychological symptoms (NPI-F) is an important aspect of carer burden and this study confirms that group intervention can moderate these, suggesting that this model of intervention has the potential to impact, at least in the short term, on the reported behavioural and psychological symptoms of people with dementia (BPSD). Whilst our study lacked a control condition, it confirms the findings of the randomised controlled study of Hébert *et al.* (2003) where reduced BPSD following a similar theoretical base to that of our study in Bologna was also noted.

Although our results are modest, one positive aspect of the carer programme in Bologna is that it reflects a starting point for developing more well defined and long-term psychosocial interventions which can follow the changing needs of families through their career in dementia (Montgomery and Kosloski 1999). In the follow-up interviews, most carers stressed the importance of being able to interact with other people in similar situations, and of having the opportunity to express their feelings and emotions. This was an important adjunct to the information they received. We do not report measures of distress (anxiety and depression) although these were taken. The group intervention had little impact on carer distress but this is not surprising as, according to the theory used in this study, moderating carer mood would require a more sustained and individualised psychosocial intervention (Brodaty *et al.* 2003). The opportunity for continued group support and individual counselling has, we suggest, the potential to moderate carer mood and if the programme is offered at the start of the family journey (Caron, Pattee and Otteson 2000) there is scope to prevent breakdown of care at home, as is demonstrated in the New York studies of individualised psychosocial intervention in family carers (Mittelman *et al.* 2004).

One source of optimism for this group intervention in Italy is that it is set within a regional policy that aspires to improve services for people with dementia and their carers, thus allowing scope for adjusting international research in psychosocial intervention in dementia and implementing this within local communities in Italy.

References

Brodaty, H., Green, A. and Graham, N. (2000) 'Alzheimer's (Disease and Related Disorders) Associations and Societies: Supporting Family Carers.' In J. O'Brien, D. Ames and A. Burns (eds) *Dementia*. London: Arnold.

Brodaty, H., Green, A. and Koschera, A. (2003) 'Meta-analysis of psychosocial interventions for caregivers of people with dementia.' *Journal of the American Geriatric Society 51*, 657–664.

Caron, W.A., Pattee, J.J. and Otteson, O.J. (2000) *Alzheimer's Disease: The Family Journey*. Plymouth: North Ridge Press.

Carver, C.S., Scheier, M.F. and Weintraub, J.K. (1989) 'Assessing coping strategies: a theoretically based approach.' *Journal of Personality and Social Psychology 56*, 267–283.

Charlesworth, G. (2001) 'Reviewing psychosocial interventions for family carers of people with dementia.' *Aging and Mental Health 5*, 104–106.

Cooke, D.D., McNally, L., Mulligan, K.T., Harrison, M.J.G. and Newman, S.P. (2001) 'Psychosocial interventions for caregivers of people with dementia: a systematic review.' *Aging and Mental Health 5*, 120–135.

Coon, D.W., Gallagher-Thompson, D. and Thompson, L.W. (eds) (2003a) *Innovative Interventions to Reduce Dementia Caregiver Distress: A Clinical Guide*. New York, NY: Springer.

Coon, D.W., Ory, M.G. and Schulz, R. (2003b) 'Family Caregivers: Enduring and Emergent Themes.' In D.W. Coon, D. Gallagher-Thompson and L.W. Thompson (eds) *Innovative Interventions to Reduce Dementia Caregiver Distress: A Clinical Guide*. New York, NY: Springer.

Cummings, J.L., Mega, M.S., Gray, K., Rosemberg-Thompson, S. and Gornbein, T. (1994) 'The neuropsychiatric inventory: comprehensive assessment of psychopathology in dementia.' *Neurology 44*, 2308–2314.

Dunkin, J. and Anderson-Hanley, C. (1998) 'Dementia caregiver burden: a review of the literature and guidelines for assessment and intervention.' *Neurology 51* (suppl.1), S53–S60.

Folstein, M.F., Folstein, S.E. and McHugh, P.R. (1975) 'Mini-mental state: a practical method for grading the cognitive state of patients for the clinician.' *Journal of Psychiatric Research 12*, 189–198.

Ford, G.R., Goode, K.T., Barrett, J.J., Harrell, L.E. and Haley, W.E. (1997) 'Gender roles and caregiving stress: an examination of subjective appraisal of specific primary stressors in Alzheimer's caregivers.' *Aging and Mental Health 1*, 158–165.

Hébert, R., Lévesque, L., Vezina, J., Lavoie, J., *et al.* (2003) 'Efficacy of a psychoeducative group program for caregivers of demented persons living at home: a randomized controlled trial.' *Journal of Gerontology Series B – Psychological and Social Sciences 58*, S58–S67.

Knight, B.G., Lutzky, S.M. and Macofsky-Urban, F. (1993) 'A meta-analytic review of interventions for caregiver distress: recommendations for future research.' *Gerontologist 33*, 240–248.

Lavoie, J.P. (1995) 'Support groups for informal caregivers don't work! Refocus the groups or the evaluations?' Canadian Journal on Aging/La Revue Canadienne du Vieillissement 14, 580–595.

Lazarus, R.S. and Folkman, S. (1984) *Stress, Coping and Appraisal*. New York, NY: Springer.

Lévesque, L., Gendron, C., Vezina, J., Hébert, R., *et al.* (2002) 'The process of a group intervention for caregivers of demented persons living at home: conceptual framework, components and characteristics.' *Aging and Mental Health 6*, 239–247.

Liberman, R.P. (1987) *Psychiatric Rehabilitation of Chronic Mental Patients*. Washington, DC: American Psychiatric Press.

Magni, E., Zanetti, O., Bianchetti, A., Binetti, G. and Trabucchi, M. (1995) 'Evaluation of an Italian educational programme for dementia caregivers: results of a smallscale pilot study.' *International Journal of Geriatric Psychiatry 10*, 569–573.

Mittelman, M.S., Roth, D.L., Haley, W. and Zarit, S.H. (2004) 'Effects of a caregiver intervention on negative caregiver appraisals of behaviour problems in patients with Alzheimer's disease: results of a randomized controlled trial.' *Journal of Gerontology: Psychological Sciences 59B*, 27–34.

Montgomery, R.J.V. and Kosloski, K.D. (1999) 'Family Caregiving: Change, Continuity and Diversity.' In R.L. Rubinstein and P. Lawton (eds) *Alzheimer's Disease and Related Dementias: Strategies in Care and Research*. New York, NY: Springer.

Murray, J. and McDaid, D. (2002) 'Carer Burden: The Difficulties and Rewards of Care-giving.' In M. Warner, S. Furnish, M. Longley and B. Lawlor (eds) *Alzheimer's Disease: Policy and Practice across Europe*. Oxford: Radcliffe.

Nobili, A., Riva, E., Tettamanti M., Lucca U., *et al.* (2004) 'The effect of a structured intervention on caregivers of patients with dementia and problem behaviours: a randomized controlled pilot study.' *Alzheimer Disease and Associated Disorders 18*, 75–82.

Novak, M. and Guest, C. (1989) 'Application of a multidimensional caregiver burden inventory.' *Gerontologist 29*, 798–803.

Ory, M.G., Hoffman, R.R., Yee, J.L., Tennstadt, S. and Schulz, R. (1999) 'Prevalence and impact of caregiving: a detailed comparison between dementia and non-dementia caregivers.' *Gerontologist* 39, 177–185.

Paykel, E.S. (1983) 'Methodological aspects of life events research.' *Journal of Psychosomatic Research* 27, 341–352.

Pusey, H. and Richards, D. (2001) 'A systematic review of the effectiveness of psychosocial interventions for carers of people with dementia.' *Aging and Mental Health 5*, 120–135.

Schulz, R. and Williamson, G.M. (1997) 'The measurement of caregiver outcomes in Alzheimer disease research.' *Alzheimer Disease and Associated Disorders 11*, 117–124.

Schulz, R., O'Brien, A.T., Bookwala, J. and Fleissner, K. (1995) 'Psychiatric and physical morbidity effects of dementia caregiving: prevalence, correlates, and causes.' *Gerontologist 35*, 771–791.

Senesi, B., Gianelli, M.V., Marcenaro, M., Polleri, A., Bonetti, R. and Molinari, R. (1999) 'Caregiving informale, stress ed adattamento emotivo nell'assistenza al paziente con demenza. I risultati di uno studio preliminare.' In G. Spinetti and A. Netti (eds) *La malattia di Alzheimer: malattia sociale*. Bologna: Edizioni Istituto Internazionale di Psichiatria e Psicoterapia.

Sica, C., Novara, C., Dorz, S. and Sanavio, E. (1997) 'Coping orientation to problem experienced (COPE): traduzione e adattamento italiano.' *Bollettino di Psicologia Applicata 233*, 23–34.

Thommesen, B., Aarsland, D., Braekhus, A., Oksengaard, A.R., Engedal, K. and Laake, K. (2002) 'The psychosocial burden on spouses of the elderly with stroke, dementia and Parkinson's disease.' *International Journal of Geriatric Psychiatry 17*, 78–84.

Vernooij-Dassen, M., Moniz-Cook, E. Woods, R., De Lepeleire, J., *et al.* (2005) 'Factors affecting timely recognition and diagnosis of dementia across Europe: from awareness to stigma.' *International Journal of Geriatric Psychiatry 20*, 377–386.

Zanetti, O., Metitieri, T., Bianchetti, A. and Trabucchi, M. (1998a) 'Effectiveness of an educational programme for demented persons' relatives.' *Archives of Gerontology and Geriatrics 6*, 531–538.

Zanetti, O., Frisoni, G.B., Bianchetti, A., Tamanza, G., Cigoli, V. and Trabucchi, M. (1998b) 'Depressive symptoms of Alzheimer caregivers are mainly due to personal rather than patient factors.' *International Journal of Geriatric Psychiatry 13*, 358–367.

Zarit, S.H. and Edwards, A.B. (1999) 'Family Caregiving: Research and Clinical Intervention.' In R.T. Woods (ed.) *Psychological Problems of Ageing*. Chichester: Wiley.

Zarit, S.H., Stephens, M.A., Townsend, A. and Greene, R. (1998) 'Stress reduction for family caregivers: effects of adult day care use.' *Journal of Gerontology 53B*, S267–S277.

Further Reading and Related References

Gianelli, M.V., Senesi, B., Molinari, L. and Polleri, A. (2000) 'How heavily does the burden of patients' cognitive impairment emotionally affect their caregivers?' Paper presented at conference on 'Non-Alzheimer Cognitive Impairment', Newcastle-upon-Tyne, 4–7 April.

PART IV

Developing Evidence-based Psychosocial Support Services

Chapter 14

The Meeting Centres Support Programme

Rose-Marie Dröes, Franka Meiland,
Jacomine de Lange, Myrra Vernooij-Dassen
and Willem van Tilburg

Overview

Over the past 15 years many types of support have been developed for people
with dementia and their carers. This has ranged from respite care, discussion
groups and informative meetings to different educational materials such as
books, information brochures and television programmes. The main drawback
of the current support offered is that it is often fragmented. To tackle these difficulties, a number of care and welfare institutions in Amsterdam combined
their support and expertise in the Meeting Centres Model, which began in
1993. The initiative was led by the Department of Psychiatry at the Vrije
Universiteit (VU) medical centre and the Valerius Foundation, a Dutch foundation that encourages innovative activities which link care and welfare for
people with mental and nervous diseases. Because of the positive experiences
and study results, the Meeting Centres Model has been disseminated to eight
other regions and 17 cities in the Netherlands. In this chapter the content of
the Meeting Centres Support Programme is discussed, together with the
theory it was based on, the research that has been conducted on it in the last ten
years, and the application in daily practice. The chapter ends with some concluding remarks about the strengths and potential limitations of the support
programme, and some factors that must be taken into account in establishing a
meeting centre.

The Meeting Centres Support Programme integrated various support activities, which have already been proven effective by research and practice, for

people with dementia and their carers (Cuijpers 1992; Dröes 1991; Dröes and van Tilburg 1996; Finnema *et al.* 2000a; De Lange *et al.* 1999; Vernooij-Dassen 1993). Carers attend informative meetings and discussion groups, and access respite care and practical help to arrange care at home and, if necessary, placement in a nursing home. People with dementia (a maximum of 15 per centre) utilise social clubs in the community centre, or centres for older people, where they participate in a variety of creative and recreational activities. Furthermore, carers and people with dementia use a weekly counselling session and a monthly meeting for all participants. A collaborative system records how the regional care and welfare institutions participate in the support programme. The small-scale, integrated and intensive nature of the support, which happens close to home, fosters a trusting relationship with the meeting centre staff. This makes it easier for carers to accept help and share the caregiving with others.

Theoretical background

The support programme was based mainly on the Adaptation-Coping Model (Dröes 1991; Dröes *et al.* 2000; Finnema *et al.* 2000b) which was derived from the coping theory of Lazarus and Folkman (1984) and the crises model of Moos and Tsu (1977). In the Adaptation-Coping Model behavioural problems in people with dementia were partly explained as reactions or (in)adequate ways of coping (naturally partly due to the dementia) with the stress caused by a number of general adaptive tasks. For example, the person may have experienced problems with:

- dealing with their disabilities

- preserving an emotional balance

- maintaining a positive self-image

- preparing for an uncertain future

- developing and maintaining social relationships

- dealing with the institutional environment and treatment procedures

- developing an adequate relationship with staff.

The programme offered people with dementia and their carers emotional support in the process of accepting the disease, in dealing with the difficult times they may face, and in their changing relationship. It also aimed to decrease feelings of stress and increase feelings of self-esteem and competence in both the person with dementia and their carer, by influencing their appraisal of their situation and their coping processes (Dröes 1996). The older people with dementia were also assisted in adapting to other problems they experienced because of their disabilities. The general goals of the support programme were:

- to inform carers about dementia and coping strategies, so that they learned to cope with the behavioural changes in the person with dementia

- to let the carer and the person with dementia experience emotional support from other people who are in the same situation

- to increase the social network of the carer and the person with dementia, and thereby increase the support of the social environment

- to give the carer some respite to reduce the burden of care

- to assist and support people with dementia in adapting to and coping with their own disabilities and deterioration, with the ultimate goal of improving the quality of their life.

Recruitment and inclusion criteria

People with mild to moderate dementia and their carers who participated in the programme were recruited via local newspapers, posters, (e.g. in general practitioners' (GPs') surgeries and pharmacies, and brochures. Selection took place on the basis of the diagnosis 'dementia syndrome' and the level of severity of the dementia. The diagnosis was always made by a medical doctor, i.e. a general practitioner, a doctor at the local psychiatric service or by a psychiatrist or neurologist in, for example, a memory clinic. A criterion for the carer was that he or she should be motivated to participate in the support programme.

Research

Research by the VU medical centre between 1994 and 1996 (in four meeting centres in the Amsterdam area; Dröes 1996; Dröes *et al.* 2000) and between 2000 and 2003 (in five other regions in the Netherlands; Dröes *et al.* 2003b) demonstrated that the combined support in meeting centres had additional value when compared with standard day care in nursing homes. People with dementia who utilised the Meeting Centres Support Programme over a longer period of time (seven months) had less behavioural and mood problems (less antisocial behaviour, inactivity and depressed behaviour in particular; delayed nursing home admission) than people who visited ordinary day care centres. Also, the strength of the carers was greater (fewer experienced burden, keeping up the care for a longer period of time and at a better level; expanding their social networks) compared to carers who visited ordinary day care. The second study also demonstrated that lone carers who participated in the Meeting Centres Support Programme developed fewer psychological and psychosomatic complaints. The costs of the integrated support were no higher than the costs of ordinary day care in nursing homes, which meant that a larger effect was achieved at the same cost.

With regard to the people with dementia who participated in the support programme it was found that the majority had four or more neuropsychiatric symptoms (as measured by the Neuropsychiatric Inventory, NPI; Cummings *et al.* 1994). Over half of the participating carers had psychological and/or psychosomatic complaints (as measured by the General Health Questionnaire; Goldberg and Hillier 1979).

People with dementia as well as their carers were very satisfied with the support and some of them (half of the people with dementia and one-third of the carers) viewed the people they met at the meeting centre as new friends. Dissatisfaction regarding the meeting centres (e.g. the furnishings) and the support programme itself (e.g. frequency of programme elements) was reported only by a small minority.

The effects of the support programme in the first study in Amsterdam (1994–1996) were largely similar to the effects found in the second implementation study (2000–2003) in six other regions of the Netherlands where new meeting centres were started. A quasi-experimental pre- and post-test control group design with two matched groups was applied to study the specific effect of the experimental programme. The matching took place on severity of dementia, the care needs of the person with dementia, and feelings of competence in the caregiver. In both studies the same ordinary day care control group was used. Measurement took place before the intervention (at baseline) and after seven months.

Application

The meeting centres offered practical, emotional, and social support for people with dementia and their carers. In this section we describe how this was achieved.

Activities for the person with dementia

In the social club, which opened on Mondays, Wednesdays and Fridays from 10 am until 4 pm, the person with dementia participated in several activities such as domestic activities (guided shopping or washing dishes), and creative activities and recreational activities, such as listening to music and reading the newspaper. In addition they could participate in psychomotor therapy three times a week (Dröes 1997a, 1997b; Dröes and Van Tilburg 1996) and could make use of the counselling hour once a week (see Figure 14.1). In the social club there were always two professional helpers present (see below).

Examples of the general care strategies used for the person with dementia were: reactivation, resocialisation and improving their affective functioning. Of course, combinations of strategies were also possible. Several emotion-oriented approaches were used, such as validation, reminiscence and reality orientation assistance.

Activities for family carers

Support strategies for caregivers varied from giving information and practical help by, for example, informative meetings and case management, to offering emotional support through discussion groups, and increasing their social network by encouraging participation in social and cultural activities. The informative meetings (in total eight to ten lectures about dementia and handling of behavioural problems) were organised once a fortnight. The discussion group also came together once a fortnight. Carers participated in it as long as they felt the need to do so. Both the informative meetings and the discussion groups lasted about two hours per meeting. The programme co-ordinator organised both groups. For the informative meetings professional speakers (e.g. a psychologist, a neurologist, a social worker, etc.) were invited to talk about specific themes. The counselling hour was held weekly by the programme co-ordinator at a fixed time. Participants visited the centre or contacted the centre by telephone. Finally, some activities were organised for the carer and the person with dementia together, such as the monthly centre meeting that was organised to adapt the programme to the needs of the participating group at that time, and recreational activities (see Figure 14.1). The staff of the programme worked together with psychiatric and psychogeriatric ambulant services, including community nursing and home care, and with the general practitioner for consultation.

Meeting Centres Support Programme

For the carer

- Informative meetings
- Discussion group

For the people with dementia

- Social club
- Psychomotor therapy

For both

- Counselling hour
- Case management
- Monthly meeting where staff and participants meet

- Recreational activities

Goal

- Education
- Emotional and social support

- Assistance and support in coping with their own deterioration

- Individual support and advice
- Practical support
- Adapting the programme to the needs of the participating group at that time
- Optimising communication between staff and participants
- Expansion of social network

Figure 14.1 The programme and its goals

Case example – Walter and Dorothy

During a visit to the GP Dorothy complained about being nervous all the time and having frequent headaches. The GP felt that she had become overburdened due to caring for her husband, whom she loved dearly and had looked after since his diagnosis of dementia. A recent added strain for both Walter and Dorothy was the deterioration of his eyesight over the past year. The GP therefore advised Dorothy to get in touch with the Meeting Centres Support Programme. It was thought that they could both receive support at the same time, since it was unlikely that either Walter or Dorothy would easily agree to part with the other during the day so that Dorothy could have traditional 'respite' such as day care.

At the meeting centre it was suggested that Walter participated in the social club three days a week, whilst Dorothy could join the carer programme that was organised one afternoon a week and receive both emotional support and information on how to cope with the daily problems she encountered in caring for her husband. As an add-on, if they both liked the meeting centre, Dorothy would also be able to have some respite on the other two days that her husband attended the centre.

Initially Walter and Dorothy had a period of getting to know what was available. Dorothy reported that she liked the small size, the relaxed atmosphere and the individual attention that the few members of staff appeared to give to the participants. She particularly felt that the opportunity to listen to classical music would be of interest to her husband, as his vision was deteriorating. The first time that she participated in the discussion group with other family members, she reported feeling a bit out of her depth, but was soon able to explain her experience of how she suffered from losing her husband bit by bit. Through this opportunity to describe what it felt like for her, she was able to experience the relief of shared support. During one psycho-educational meeting, it dawned on her that the somatic complaints that she sometimes experienced were connected with the sorrow and the fear of losing her husband.

When Walter attended the meeting centre without his wife, Dorothy filled her time with cleaning the house and shopping. She initially reported that she found it difficult to do things that were just for herself, since she would think of her husband and feel guilty. However, when she attended the meeting centre, she had the opportunity to have a cup of coffee with others after the discussion group. Dorothy began to have coffee with another woman of her own age who also had a husband with dementia. Over time they gradually became friends. In the spring, when the new activity agenda at the community centre had been announced, they decided to do a course in flower arranging. They had great fun and after every meeting they would have a cup of tea or coffee together at the social club. Her husband was observed to beam with happiness when he heard her cheerful voice, 'She is still the best!'

Conclusion and implications for future research

The 'added value' aspect of the Meeting Centres Model was that it combated fragmentation by offering a broad and integrated support programme for people with mild to moderate dementia, as well as for their carers, in an easily accessible location (community centre and centre for the elderly), by a small and permanent professional team (a programme co-ordinator, an activity therapist and a nursing assistant). This rendered the service, especially in the early stages of dementia (and for younger people with dementia), less threatening than the standard day care offered in institutions such as nursing homes and homes for the elderly in the Netherlands. As a result help was requested at an earlier stage.

Research has shown that behavioural disorders of people with mild to moderate dementia, overburdening of carers, and psychological and

psychosomatic complaints in lone carers could be partly prevented by participation in the Meeting Centres Support Programme.

To stimulate national implementation, the conditions of successful
practice were investigated by the Department of Psychiatry at the VU medical
centre in Amsterdam, in conjunction with the University Medical Centre St
Radboud in Nijmegen and the Trimbos Institute in Utrecht. This study
showed that implementation in other regions did not lead to major changes in
the programme design or execution, or in changes in the target group (people
with dementia and their carers). In other words, the Meeting Centres Support
Programme represented a well-defined facility bridging care and welfare. All
elements of the programme were offered in easily accessible locations by a
small professional staff and volunteers. With regard to the people with
dementia taking part, the majority of them showed behavioural and psychological symptoms, over half of the carers had psychological and/or
psychosomatic complaints.

Factors that helped and factors that hindered the implementation of the
Meeting Centres Support Programme in six regions of the Netherlands were
assessed on the basis of a theoretical model that was designed specifically for
this study. The model classified these facilitators and barriers at the micro-
(primary process), meso- (social context and organisation) and macro-levels
(structures, legislation) during three phases of the implementation process: the
preparation phase, the introduction phase and the continuation phase. A diversity of facilitators and barriers were found for different phases of implementation. Factors that were important in all phases were: motivated people (key
figures, innovators, personnel); cooperation with other organisations (regarding referrals, appropriateness of care, discharge, cooperation on parts of the
support programme such as discussion groups, informative meetings); a
proactive public relations strategy to recruit the target group (i.e. people with
mild to moderate dementia and carers in need of support); and the availability
of funds. With the growing numbers of older people in the coming decades,
this last factor will be increasingly important to safeguard the continuation of
this kind of support which links care and welfare.

Acknowledgements

Parts of this chapter were published previously in Dröes et al. (2002), Dröes et
al. (2003a) and Dröes, Meiland and van Tilburg (2006).

References

Cuijpers, P. (1992) 'De effecten van ondersteuningsgroepen voor verzorg(st)ers van dementerende ouderen thuis: een literatuuroverzicht.' [The effects of support groups for carers of dementing elderly people at home: a literature review.] *Tijdschrift voor Gerontologie en Geriatrie 23*, 12–17.

Cummings, J.L., Mega, M., Gray, K., Rosenberg-Thompson, S., Carusi, D.A. and Gornbein, J. (1994) 'The neuropsychiatric inventory: comprehensive assessment of psychopathology in dementia.' *Neurology 44*, 2308–2314.

Dröes, R.M. (1991) 'In beweging: over psychosociale hulpverlening aan demente ouderen.' [In movement: on psychosocial care for the demented elderly.] Nijkerk: Intro.

Dröes, R.M. (1996) 'Amsterdamse ontmoetingscentra; een nieuwe vorm van ondersteuning voor mensen met dementie en hun verzorgers.' [Amsterdam meeting centres; a new form of support for people with dementia and their carers.] Amsterdam: Thesis Publishers.

Dröes, R.M. (1997a) 'Psychomotor Group Therapy for Demented Patients in the Nursing Home.' In B. Miesen and G. Jones (eds) *Care-giving in Dementia*. London: Routledge.

Dröes, R.M. (1997b) *Beweeg met ons mee! Een activeringsprogramma in groepsverband* [Let's move together! An activation programme for groups of people with dementia.] Utrecht: Elsevier/De Tijdstroom.

Dröes, R.M. and van Tilburg, W. (1996) 'Amélioration du comportement agressif par des activités psychomotrices.' [Improvement of aggressive behaviour by psychomotor activities.] *L'Année Gérontologique 10*, 471–482.

Dröes, R.M., Breebaart, E., Ettema, T.P., van Tilburg, W. and Mellenbergh, G.J. (2000) 'The effect of integrated family support versus day care only on behavior and mood of patients with dementia.' *International Psychogeriatrics 12*, 99–116.

Dröes, R.M., Breebaart, E., Ettema, T.P., Meiland, F.J.M., Mellenbergh, G.J. and van Tilburg, W. (2002) 'Effect of Meeting Centers Support Program on Persons with Dementia and Their Carers.' In S. Andrieu and J.P. Aquino (eds) *Research and Practice in Alzheimer's Disease: Family and Professional Carers' Findings Lead to Action*. New York, NY: Springer.

Dröes, R.M., Meiland, F.J.M., de Lange, J., Vernooij-Dassen, M.J.F.J. and van Tilburg, W. (2003a) 'The meeting centres support programme: an effective way of supporting people with dementia who live at home and their carers.' *Dementia: The International Journal of Social Research and Practice 2*, 426–432.

Dröes, R.M., Meiland, F.J.M., Schmitz, M.J., Vernooij-Dassen, M.J.F.J., *et al.* (2003b) *Implementatie Model Ontmoetingscentra; een onderzoek naar de voorwaarden voor succesvolle landelijke implementatie van ontmoetingscentra voor mensen met dementie en hun verzorgers. Eindrapport.* [Implementation Meeting Centers Model; a study into the conditions of successful national implementation of meeting centers for people with dementia and their carers. Final report.] Amsterdam: Department of Psychiatry, VU Medical Center.

Dröes, R.M., Meiland, F.J.M. and van Tilburg, W. (2006) 'The Meeting Centers Support Programme Model for Persons with Dementia and Their Carers: Aims, Methods and Research.' In B. Miesen and G.M.M. Jones (eds) *Care-Giving in Dementia: Research and Applications*, Vol. 4. London: Routledge.

Finnema, E.J., Dröes, R.M., Ribbe, M.W. and van Tilburg, W. (2000a) 'The effects of emotion-oriented approaches in the care for persons suffering from dementia: a review of the literature.' *International Journal of Geriatric Psychiatry 15*, 141–161.

Finnema, E., Dröes, R.M., Ribbe, M. and van Tilburg, W. (2000b) 'A review of psychosocial models in psychogeriatrics: implications for care and research.' *Alzheimer Disease and Associated Disorders 14*, 68–80.

Goldberg, D.P. and Hillier, V.F. (1979) 'A scaled version of the general health questionnaire.' *Psychological Medicine 9*, 139–145.

De Lange, J., Dröes, R.M., Finnema, E. and van der Kooij, C.H. (1999) 'Aansluiting bij de belevingswereld; effectieve zorg voor dementerenden.' [Attuning to the experience; effective care for people with dementia.] *Alzheimer Magazine 12*, 16–19.

Lazarus, R.S. and Folkman, S. (1984) *Stress, Appraisal and Coping*. New York, NY: Springer.

Moos, R.H. and Tsu, V.D. (1977) 'The Crisis of Physical Illness: An Overview.' In R.H. Moos (ed.) *Coping with Physical Illness*. Oxford: Plenum.

Vernooij-Dassen, M.J.F.J. (1993) 'Dementie en thuiszorg: een onderzoek naar determinanten van het competentiegevoel van centrale verzorgers en het effect van professionele interventie.' [Dementia and home care: a study into the determinants of the feeling of competence of central carers and the effectiveness of professional intervention.] Amsterdam/Lisse: Swets & Zeitlinger.

Further reading and related references

Dröes, R.M., Boelens-Van der Knoop, E.J., Bos, J., Meihuizen, L., *et al.* (2006) 'Quality of life in dementia in perspective: an explorative study of variations in opinions among people with dementia and their professional caregivers, and in literature.' *Dementia: The International Journal of Social Research and Practice 5*, 533–558.

Dröes, R.M., Meiland, F.J.M., Schmitz, M.J., Boerema, I., *et al.* (2004) 'Variations in meeting centers for people with dementia and their carers: results of a multi-centre implementation study.' *Archives of Geriatrics and Gerontology 9*, 127–148.

Dröes, R.M., Meiland, F.J.M., Schmitz, M. and van Tilburg, W. (2004) 'Effect of combined support for people with dementia and carers versus regular day care on behaviour and mood of persons with dementia: results from a multi-centre implementation study.' *International Journal of Geriatric Psychiatry 19*, 1–12.

Dröes, R.M., Meiland, F.J.M., Schmitz, M. and van Tilburg, W. (2006) 'Effect of the meeting centres support programme on informal carers of people with dementia: results from a multi-centre study.' *Aging and Mental Health 10*, 112–124.

Meiland, F.J.M., Dröes, R.M., de Lange, J. and Vernooij-Dassen, M.J.F.J. (2005) 'Facilitators and barriers in the implementation of the meeting centres model for people with dementia and their carers.' *Health Policy 71*, 243–253.

Chapter 15

Personalised Disease Management for People with Dementia

The Primary Carer Support Programme

Myrra Vernooij-Dassen, Maud Graff
and Marcel Olde Rikkert

Overview

This chapter describes an early support programme that is targeted at the primary carer (usually a spouse or child) of the person with dementia living at home. The programme is seen as an 'early intervention' in that it is a systematic, proactive approach directed at primary carers who provide support to the person with dementia, but who often need support themselves (Vernooij-Dassen and Dautzenberg 2003). It also follows a 'disease management' care protocol, where systematic integrated care within available resources (Ellrodt *et al.* 1997) aims to minimise the bio-psychosocial consequences of the disease and its disclosure. Thus co-ordinated care is not simply a reaction to a crisis, but is focused on the duality of the personal consequences of the disease (dementia) alongside the 'caregiving career' (Aneshensel *et al.* 1995). The management of dementia requires practitioners from a variety of disciplines to use a range of treatment and support methods with people with dementia and also with their primary carers. These can sometimes include biomedical care (including the use of medication) but more often than not some forms of psychosocial care such as active listening and emotional support is an important requirement. The programme described in this chapter is set within a disease management perspective, but focuses on psychosocial support for the primary carer. First, the theoretical and practical background to the programme and the evidence for it are summarised. Second, the programme in practice is described and illustrated. Third, its strengths and potential limitations are considered. Finally, we examine the potential for this programme to be set within a broader disease management protocol, involving multidisciplinary staff in the support of people with dementia and their primary carers.

Rationale

Background and evidence for the primary carer support programme

A prerequisite of this programme is that practitioners who support people with dementia need to accept that it is also their task to support primary carers. General practitioners (GPs) may indeed accept that they need to address the problems of primary carers of people with dementia (van Hout *et al.* 2000). However, in practice, some studies suggest that in the absence of medical complaints only a quarter are proactive in paying attention to primary carers (Simon and Kendrich 2001). Even direct educational interventions that are aimed at helping GPs to consider the needs of family carers may not always result in changes in their actual behaviour (Downs *et al.* 2002). Often they may want to do something to help families, but may not know what to do. There is some evidence that GPs may only be prepared to engage in early detection of dementia if there are early responsive management solutions available (Iliffe, Wilcock and Haworth 2006). Other practitioners will also need the skills and confidence to work with people at early stages and these are possessed by or transferable to many levels:

> Early diagnosis allows individual patients and their carers to be informed and appropriate management instigated and so professionals need to be equipped to help people over longer periods, starting with planning for the future. Professionals will be expected to facilitate preliminary introduction to appropriate agencies and support networks for both people with dementia and their families since these can relieve the significant psychological distress that carers may experience. (Iliffe and Manthorpe 2004, p.5)

Several programmes have been developed to support primary carers of people with dementia, such as respite or short break care (Gaugler *et al.* 2003), telephone support (Goodman and Pynoos 1990) and psycho-educational interventions (Herbert *et al.* 2003). The most effective of these uses an individualised approach, in which interventions are tailored to the specific needs of carers and the professionals (Acton and Kang 2001; Vernooij-Dassen *et al.*

2000, see Brodaty, Green and Koschera 2003 for a review). Dementia care is one area of practice in any discipline where an individualised approach is essential:

> Change is the core issue in dementia care, with multiple pathways of change that need to be understood at clinical and organisational levels. Practitioners and people with dementia are engaged in managing emotional, social and physical risks, making explicit risk management a potentially important component of dementia care. (Iliffe *et al.* 2005, p.1)

One primary carer programme that uses a 'disease management' protocol is the family support programme developed by Bengtson and Kuypers (1985). This programme begins by systematically evaluating the concerns and problems experienced by the carer and then developing family-specific care plans, the effects of which are then evaluated. The programme meets many of the principles of 'disease management' in that it provides a systematic and co-ordinated approach to using available resources in order to improve the quality of care in long-term conditions (see, for example, Vickrey *et al.* 2006). This systematic framework for informing case or care management attempts to maximise available resources whilst at the same time providing the flexibility to develop plans that are individualised in conjunction with the person with dementia and the carer. This differentiates it from other more traditional forms of disease management, where the focus is on the disease and the patient rather than on the person with the long-term condition and their carer (Vernooij-Dassen and Moniz-Cook 2005). The 'disease management' programme described in this chapter, the 'primary carer support programme', was derived from the family support programme of Bengston and Kuypers (1985) in the USA.

We start this chapter with a brief outline of the theoretical underpinnings of the programme, the adaptations that we made to the original family support programme and the evidence base for this primary carer support programme.

Theoretical background and evidence

The theoretical basis for this programme lies within the problem-solving literature. Two basic theoretical positions from the social sciences have been combined. First there is the symbolic interactionist perspective (Marshall 1986), which contends that people depend on and influence each other. Here this is translated to mean that the person with dementia will inevitably influence the primary carer. This has a strong empirical basis (Burns and Rabins 2000) and there is further evidence that the more general social context may also strongly influence the person with dementia (Opie, Rosewarne and O'Connor 1999). The second theoretical perspective relates to the meaning that a person may attribute to a particular situation. For example, a carer may act upon his or her perception of a situation, and this perception may influence the intervention used. Interventions with carers of people with dementia were derived from the stress–appraisal–coping model of Pearlin and Schooler (1978), and within this context there is some support for this second theoretical perspective. The primary carer support programme we developed therefore focuses particularly on the meaning or perception attached to a situation by the primary carer, with intervention targeted at altering this view if necessary.

The family support programme of Bengtson and Kuypers (1985) was adapted and shortened to improve its use with primary carers of people with dementia living at home. The programme can be used by professionals such as GPs, home helps, district nurses, occupational therapists, and those working in older people's services and mental health services, all of whom help to address the problems of carers looking after a person with dementia living at home. The original programme was applied by trained and supervised home helps and was effective in strengthening the sense of competence of female carers living with people with dementia, and in delaying the admission of the person with dementia to residential or nursing home care (Vernooij-Dassen *et al.* 2000).

Description and application of the primary carer support programme

The programme aims to strengthen the primary carer's sense of competence by reducing the negative consequences of caring; to strengthen carer satisfaction with his or her own performance as a carer; and to strengthen carer satisfaction with the person receiving care. 'Sense of competence' refers to the capacity of the primary carer to feel that they are supporting the person with dementia (Vernooij-Dassen, Felling and Persoon 1996). Sense of competence represents three domains of systematic evaluation of carer need, which then allows the development of family-specific care planning. Box 15.1 shows the three domains and the types of questions that are asked of carers. It also illustrates some of the strategies that were used by home helps to address these problems, using available health and social care resources, during the development and evaluation of the programme. Problem or 'need' identification allows targeting on the 'real life' concerns of the carer and helps prevent crises. It offers suggestions for both emotional and practical support in early and also later stages of caregiving.

Box 15.1 Questions for carers and potential strategies

Areas of carer need: Short Sense of Competence Questionnaire (SSCQ; Vernooij-Dassen et al. 1999)

Domain 1: Consequences of caring for the personal life of the carer

- I feel that the present situation with my...does not allow me as much privacy as I'd like.
- I feel stressed between trying to give to my...as well as deal with other family responsibilities, job, etc.

Strategy for management: organise additional professional support (see case example Eleanor)

Domain 2: Satisfaction with one's own performance as a carer

- I feel strained in my interaction with my...
- I wish that my...and I had a better relationship.

Strategy for management: open a dialogue regarding expectations, resources and conflicts (see case example Hannah)

Domain 3: Satisfaction with the person with dementia as a recipient of care

- I feel that my...behaves the way s/he does to have her/his own way.
- I feel that my...behaves the way s/he does to annoy me.
- I feel that my... tries to manipulate me.

Strategy for management: clarify the relationship between the person's behaviour and the dementia syndrome (see case example Ingrid)

Application of the programme

Application involves training support workers (in this case home helps) within a framework of real people and situations that are found in daily practice. The practitioners use systematic evaluation, including the Sense of Competence checklist (Vernooij-Dassen et al. 1999) to identify a problem or area of need and use problem-solving strategies. Problem identification, decision-making strategies and solutions or the best way forward are essentially collaborative and reached in consultation with the primary carer. However, within this collaborative framework the practitioner is also strongly influenced by the theoretical framework of the programme (i.e. the potential for cognitive/appraisal restructuring) and the availability of local resources for support, which are included in the problem-solving consultation. One example of the former involves assisting the carer to see if the burden of caring can be shared, whilst an example of the latter involves providing knowledge and opportunity for the carer to access the right help for a particular problem. Goals within each intervention should also be broken down into small entities, which should be clear and achievable. GPs can be asked, for example, to assist the carer to get a good night's sleep, or occupational therapists can be asked about disability and mobility aids and so forth. Our experience suggests that even when only small and limited goals are achieved, an unbearable situation may change into one where there is still some hope and pleasure in life. Thus, the primary carer can be guided in specific situations and both emotional and practical support can be identified as needs to be met. Emotional support includes offering an opportunity to express and discuss feelings and problems. Practical support can be provided by finding feasible solutions to problems and by providing help.

A final aim of the primary carer support programme is to empower carers who can then realise their wishes and avoid things that they do not wish to do. Through this process of mobilising carers' strengths, it is anticipated that exhaustion or burnout may be prevented.

Case studies

The cases that follow illustrate how carers' needs may be met using the programme described.

Case example – Eleanor

Eleanor cares for her mother who has early dementia. She has a part-time job and a one-year-old grandson. She feels as if she no longer has a life of her own. She wants to care for her mother but she also wants to assist her daughter and enjoy her grandson by looking after him once a week. She loves her job and her dilemma relates to privacy and an independent life of her own.

Emotional support
Demonstrate empathy and explore by actively listening to her wishes regarding a 'life of her own'.

Practical support
Try to find practical ways to fulfil her wish about 'a life of her own' through problem solving and using knowledge of available resources, such as arranging day care or home care that will be acceptable and

enjoyable for her mother by relating to her interests and previous activities.

Case example – Hannah

Hannah has been caring for her husband with dementia for three months. She feels exhausted and thinks that her relationship with her husband has deteriorated. Her daughter Angela persuades her to visit Aunt Elizabeth for two days while Angela looks after her father. She visits Elizabeth and enjoys her break very much. However, when she returns home she finds that her husband's condition has worsened and the home is in a mess. She feels guilty, as she now believes that she should have stayed at home and looked after him herself. The community nurse considers that an aim of her support will be to improve Hannah's interaction and relationship with her husband and to reduce her feelings of guilt.

Emotional support

Empathic listening with Hannah provides the opportunity to relieve feelings of distress. Cognitive restructuring would also involve discussion about whether her expectations of herself were what she might expect of others, or whether they were, in fact, somewhat unachievable: assisting her to consider what she *can* do, rather than what she feels she *ought* to do.

Practical support

Make it possible for her to do what she can, and discuss the possibilities of additional help, including regular breaks.

Case example – Ingrid

Ingrid has worked for several years as a home help for the Jenson family as Mrs Jenson is disabled following a stroke. She notices that Mr Jenson is no longer able to visit his daughter because he cannot manage to travel alone by bus. She also observes that Mrs Jenson is very irritated by her husband's behaviour, especially when he forgets things he promised to do, such as buying milk. She thinks he is cheating on her. What can Ingrid do to help Mrs Jenson?

Emotional support

Ingrid listens to Mrs Jenson's concerns about her husband and asks her what she thinks the reason is for his behaviour. She suggests that Mrs Jenson asks her husband to visit the GP and, if he will not, that Mrs

Jenson contact the GP herself. She tells Mrs Jenson that this seems a good way to help deal with her anxieties.

Practical support

Ingrid offers to make the appointment with the GP and to arrange transport to the appointment as Mrs Jenson finds it difficult to travel on her own. She also suggests that Mrs Jenson makes a list of her concerns as she finds it difficult to talk with professionals.

As with most problem-solving approaches, each intervention strategy needs to be evaluated and revised, based on the outcome, so that new plans can be made if necessary to adequately address the carer's problems or needs, or to ensure long-term effects.

What works for whom and what is needed to maximise outputs?

The principal advantages of this proactive primary carer support programme are its potential for systematic and integrated carer-specific evaluation, and for collaborative support that is based on need and available resources. It is therefore valuable in a disease management protocol of care or care pathway for dementia. The programme has a strong theoretical and empirical base and has been effective in empowering carers by, for example, strengthening their sense of competence. This in turn has delayed some possible admissions to residential or nursing homes (Vernooij-Dassen *et al.* 2000). It can be carried out by a variety of practitioners, such as GPs, geriatricians, home helps, district nurses and occupational therapists, and can be incorporated into routine care. For example, occupational therapists can assess specific problems at home and respond to these by providing practical and emotional support whilst assisting primary carers to maximise their relative's capacities by adapting aspects of their home, such as by making adjustments to cookers or furniture. Furthermore, the programme encourages collaboration between practitioners. In this programme the home helps reported feeling better able to deal with some of the difficult situations that they encountered when providing support to people with dementia and their families. This programme reflects an opportunity for practitioners to embrace the challenge of 'doing something' and not effectively abandoning people and families due to negative attitudes or feelings of helplessness about supporting people with dementia and their carers.

This intervention reflects a proactive focused programme on prevention (i.e. disease management). One significant difficulty is that such programmes with demonstrated effectiveness are not easy to maintain in daily practice. Implementation usually requires special efforts, such as supervision and support for the practitioner, to enable systematic evaluation on a routine basis, and to assist the development of realistic goals which can be reflected on and redefined on an ongoing basis. Although the programme may not require a high standard of professional qualifications (the original study involved 42 home helps), it does require motivation, creativity, communication skills and knowledge of the local situation. Therefore all disciplines need to be engaged in this type of support programme, and they need to demonstrate motivation and 'person-centred' abilities. We have noted elsewhere that assessment of the need for support should start early on, such as when the diagnosis of dementia is disclosed (Derksen *et al.* 2006) and identification of possible stressors and a carer's willingness to take on this role can be discussed in counselling and information-giving opportunities.

Another problem for all individualised case-specific interventions is the absence of standardised 'cookbook' solutions for every situation. The carer may require broad abilities among practitioners to identify a wide range of solutions – and in some ways it may be seen as a cooking guide for creative cooks! Indeed, an aspiration for standardised programmes may be unrealistic since complex problems do not often have standard solutions (Grol 2001).

While the programme was successful for many, there were some carers who did not benefit. We re-examined the research data to explore what might be the common factors, and for whom and why the programmes were successful or otherwise. This analysis was based on home helps' diary records of their activities that generated hypotheses for subgroup analysis. We found that male carers preferred breaks or forms of respite care and would choose to leave the house rather than taking the opportunity to talk with the home help. Women who were not sharing the home with the person with dementia did not make use of emotional support such as talking to the home helps. In both these situations there was usually little contact between the home help and primary carer, and only one component, i.e. practical support, was provided. Interestingly, this practical support was not enough to strengthen the carers' sense of competence. Therefore, in order to enhance disease management, it is important that we explore the essential ingredients of effectiveness of the programme. What actually enhanced a sense of competence in primary carers remains unclear. Future research may also need to examine our impressions that this programme enhances job satisfaction and feelings of competence for the home helps.

Conclusion

Throughout Europe, in common with research undertaken in the USA, care-givers of people with dementia, especially spouses and partners, often show high levels of psychological distress or burden (Manthorpe and Moriarty 2007, p.236). Interventions for carers where outcomes are positive are likely to be achieved by multidimensional interventions that are individually tailored to their needs (Woods *et al.* 2003). The primary carer programme is a problem-solving, crisis preventive, method which offers emotional and practical support. It can be delivered through a wide range of routine activities. It can enhance hope and empowerment in carers, and may reduce the likelihood of admission to residential and nursing homes of the person with dementia. However, it is dependent on the personal qualities of practitioners and also the primary carer. Carers who do not live with the person with dementia appear only to want practical support at this stage but this is highly valued when it is tailored to individual circumstances.

References

Acton, G.J. and Kang, J. (2001) 'Interventions to reduce the burden of caregiving for an adult with dementia: a meta-analysis.' *Research in Nursing and Health 24*, 349–360.

Aneshensel, C.S., Pearlin, L.I., Mullan, J.T., Zarit, S.H. and Whitlatch, C.J. (1995) *Profiles in Caregiving: The Unexpected Carer.* San Diego, CA: Academic Press.

Bengtson, V.L. and Kuypers, J. (1985) 'The Family Support Cycle: Psychosocial Issues in the Aging Family.' In J.M.A. Munnichs, E. Olbrich, P. Mussen and P.G. Coleman (eds) *Life-span and Change in a Gerontological Perspective.* New York, NY: Academic Press.

Brodaty, H., Green, A. and Koschera, A. (2003) 'Meta-analysis of psychosocial intervention for caregivers of people with dementia.' *Journal of American Geriatrics Society 51*, 675–664.

Burns, A. and Rabins, P. (2000) 'Carer burden in dementia.' *International Journal of Geriatric Psychiatry 15*, S9–S13.

Derksen, E., Vernooij-Dassen, M., Scheltens, P. and Olde Rikkert, M. (2006) 'A model for the diagnosis of dementia.' *Dementia 5*, 462–468.

Downs, M., Clibbens, R., Rae, C., Cook, A. and Woods, R. (2002) 'What do general practitioners tell people with dementia and their families about the condition? A survey of experiences in Scotland.' *Dementia 1*, 47–58.

Ellrodt, G., Cook, D.L., Lee, J., Cho, M., Hundt, D. and Weingarten, S. (1997) 'Evidence based disease management.' *Journal of the American Medical Association 278*, 1687–1692.

Gaugler, J.E., Jarrott, S.E., Zarit, S.H., Stephens, M.A., Townsend, A. and Greene, R. (2003) 'Adult day service use and reductions in caregiving hours: effects on stress and psychosocial well-being for dementia caregivers.' *International Journal of Geriatric Psychiatry 18*, 55–62.

Goodman, C.C. and Pynoos, J. (1990) 'A model telephone information and support programme for caregivers of Alzheimer's patients.' *Gerontologist 30*, 399–404.

Grol, R. (2001) 'Improving the quality of medical care: building bridges among professional pride, payer profit, and patient satisfaction.' *Journal of the American Medical Association 286*, 2407–2412.

Herbert, R., Levesque, L., Vezina, J., Lavoie, J., *et al.* (2003) 'Efficacy of a psychoeducative group program for caregivers of demented persons living at home: a randomized controlled trial.' *Journal of Gerontology Series B – Psychological and Social Science, 58*, S58–S67.

Iliffe, S. and Manthorpe, J. (2004) 'The recognition of and response to dementia in primary care: lessons for professional development.' *Learning in Health and Social Care 3*, 5–16.

Iliffe, S., De Lepeleire, J., van Hout, H., Kenny, G., *et al.* (2005) 'Understanding obstacles to the recognition of and response to dementia in different European countries: a modified focus group approach using multinational, multi-disciplinary expert groups.' *Aging and Mental Health 9*, 1–6.

Iliffe, S., Wilcock, J. and Haworth, D. (2006) 'Delivering psychosocial interventions for people with dementia in primary care: jobs or skills?' *Dementia 5*, 327–338.

Manthorpe, J. and Moriarty, J. (2007) 'Models from Other Countries: Social Work with People with Dementia and Their Caregivers.' In C. Cox (ed.) *Dementia and Social Work Practice*. New York, NY: Springer.

Marshall, V.W. (1986) 'Dominant and Emerging Paradigms in the Social Psychology of Aging.' In V.W. Marshall (ed.) *Later Life: The Social Psychology of Aging*. Beverly Hills, CA: Sage.

Opie, J., Rosewarne, R. and O'Connor, D.W. (1999) 'The efficacy of psychosocial approaches to behaviour disorders in dementia: a systematic review.' *Australian and New Zealand Journal of Psychiatry 33*, 789–799.

Pearlin, L.I. and Schooler, A. (1978) 'The structure of coping.' *Journal of Health and Social Behaviour 19*, 2–21.

Simon, C. and Kendrich, T. (2001) 'Informal carers and the role of general practitioners and district nurses.' *British Journal of General Practice 52*, 655–657.

van Hout, H., Vernooij-Dassen, M., Bakker, K., Blom, M. and Grol, R. (2000) 'General practitioners on dementia: tasks, practices and obstacles.' *Patient Education and Counselling 39*, 219–225.

Vernooij-Dassen, M. and Dautzenberg, M. (2003) 'Collaboration between Lay and Professional Care.' In R. Jones, N. Britten, L. Culpepper, D.A. Gass, *et al.* (eds) *Textbook of Primary Medical Care*. Oxford: Oxford University Press.

Vernooij-Dassen, M. and Moniz-Cook, E. (2005) 'Editorial.' *Dementia: The International Journal of Social Research and Practice 4*, 163–169.

Vernooij-Dassen, M., Felling, A.J.A. and Persoon, J.M.G. (1996) 'Predictors of sense of competence in primary caregivers of demented persons.' *Social Science and Medicine 43*, 41–49.

Vernooij-Dassen, M., Felling, E., Brummelkamp, M., Dautzenberg, G., van den Bosch, R. and Grol, R. (1999) 'Short sense of competence questionnaire (SSCQ): measuring the caregiver's sense of competence.' *Journal of the American Geriatrics Society 47*, 256–257.

Vernooij-Dassen, M.J.F.J., Lamers, C., Bor, J., Felling, A.J.A. and Grol, R. (2000) 'Prognostic factors of effectiveness of a support programme for caregivers of dementia patients.' *International Journal of Aging and Human Development 51*, 259–274.

Vickrey, B., Mittman, B., Connor, K.I., Pearson, M.L., *et al.* (2006) 'The effect of a disease management intervention on quality and outcomes of dementia.' *Annals of Internal Medicine 145*, 713–726.

Woods, R., Moniz-Cook, E., Iliffe, S., Campion, P., *et al.* (2003) 'Dementia: issues in early recognition and intervention in primary care.' *Journal of the Royal Society of Medicine 96*, 320–323.

Further Reading and Related References

Moniz-Cook, E. and Vernooij-Dassen, M. (2005) 'DIADEM: European Variations in Diagnosis and Post-diagnosis Support for People with Dementia.' In P. Dorenlot (ed.) *Supporting and Caring for People with Early Stage Dementia: Challenges, Practice and Perspectives*. Paris: Fondation Médéric Alzheimer.

Vernooij-Dassen, M. and Olde Rikkert, M.G.M. (2004) 'Personal disease management in dementia care.' *International Journal of Geriatric Psychiatry 51*, 259–274.

Vernooij-Dassen, M., Huygen, F., Felling, A. and Persoon, J. (1995) 'Home care for dementia patients.' *Journal of the American Geriatric Society 43*, 456–457.

Vernooij-Dassen, M., Moniz-Cook, E.D., Woods, B., de Lepeleire, J., *et al.* (2005) 'Factors affecting timely recognition and diagnosis of dementia across Europe: from awareness to stigma.' *International Journal of Geriatric Psychiatry 9*, 1–6.

Chapter 16

Carer Interventions in the Voluntary Sector

Georgina Charlesworth, Joanne Halford,
Fiona Poland and Susan Vaughan

Overview

Voluntary and charitable organisations have an important role to play in providing supportive, non-stigmatising, user-friendly services for carers. This chapter provides theoretical background to social support, and describes two different UK examples of support interventions for carers of people with dementia where voluntary organisations are the service providers. The first example is of a group educational programme and the second is a befriending scheme. Common to each example is a desire for carers to be supported in a holistic way, with access to emotional, informational and instrumental support, within a context of respecting the 'personhood' of both the carer and the person with dementia. Both examples include vignettes showing how support through voluntary sector interventions can make a real difference to carers of people with dementia.

Social support theory and practice

Cowen (1982) defined social support as 'informal interpersonal help with emotional problems' (p.385). Around the same time, House (1981) conceptualised social support in terms of content, or functions, suggesting dimensions of emotional, informational and instrumental support. Kahn and Antonucci (1980) combined social role and social support theories to propose the life course social support model.

By the mid-1980s, social support was being reconceptualised, with Thoits (1986) framing social support as 'coping assistance'. Heller, Swindle and Dusenbury (1986) moved away from the language of 'problems' to 'needs', defining social support as 'any informal human interaction that meets psychological needs or which helps individuals cope with adversity' (p.466). Psychological needs were seen as including: attachment needs (a close relationship that would allow nurturance, unconditional assistance and safety); social integration needs (a sense of belonging); social validation needs (recognition of identity and competence); and need for guidance (advice and information). In his book *Social Therapy* Milne (1999) brought together previous definitions as follows:

> Social support…refers to the provision of informal help in order to try and meet someone's psychological needs… It consists structurally of informational, practical and emotional assistance (e.g. sympathetically listening to a neighbour) and companionship. (Milne 1999, p.4)

It has been suggested that emotional, informational and practical (instrumental) dimensions of social support can each be related to a different mechanism of change (Barker and Pistrang 2002; Hogan, Linden and Najarian 2002; Noon 1999). More specifically, emotional support that involves verbal and non-verbal communication of caring and concern is believed to reduce distress by restoring self-esteem and permitting the expression of feelings, whereas informational support (provision of information to be used as a guide) is believed to enhance perceptions of control by reducing confusion and providing people with strategies to cope with their difficulties.

Example 1: Positive Caring Programme

The Positive Caring Programme aimed to meet carers' needs for information about living with dementia through group psycho-educational meetings provided by Alzheimer's Society branch workers. Typical of information and education sessions described in research literature (see Briggs and Askham 1999), the programme consisted of six weekly sessions, each lasting approximately two hours, and covering a different topic each week. Information was provided on the caring role, dementia, benefits, the law, local services and practical care management advice (e.g. moving, handling and equipment). Time was also spent developing carers' stress management skills such as relaxation and communication. Efforts were made to provide ongoing support for carers by building up good relationships and maintaining contact beyond the end of the group.

Case example – Betty and Jim

After 50 years of happy marriage, Betty began to notice changes in her husband Jim's behaviour. Over the previous two years he had started to become confused and forgetful. He was finding it increasingly difficult to recall recent events. He was becoming quite anxious, and Betty was too. At first she hoped Jim would get better, but things only got worse, so she went to their family doctor. Jim was referred to see a psychiatrist. That was the start of a lot of questions and tests. Eventually Jim was given the diagnosis of Alzheimer's disease. At the time Betty did not have much of an opportunity to discuss her husband's problems, and afterwards she found she had lots of questions in her mind. Some time later another family doctor in the practice suggested that she get in touch with the Alzheimer's Society. She found out about the Positive Caring Programme being run by her local branch, but initially thought she wouldn't be able to attend as she didn't want to leave Jim alone. The group co-ordinator told her about a sitting service that could be arranged where a careworker would spend time with Jim at home. The service was arranged and Betty attended the group. Even after the first session, she felt as if a weight had been lifted from her shoulders. At last she was getting answers to all the questions she had never had the opportunity to ask. She was able to share her experiences with other carers and learn that she wasn't the only one who felt frustrated and angry with their loved one. She found out about different kinds of allowances and suggestions for organising finances. She learned ways of understanding and coping with her husband's behaviour, and also ways to look after herself. At the end of the course she commented, 'The whole course has been very helpful. I cannot believe how much it has helped me cope with our situation.'

An evaluation of the programme was carried out between September 2001 and April 2002 (Halford 2002) with a total of 24 attendees from courses in four different locations within East Anglia (Mid-Suffolk, Norwich, Huntingdon and Ipswich). Carers were predominantly female (n = 17), with one in three participants being wives (a quarter daughters and a quarter husbands). Carers' mean age was 68 years (range 43 to 81 years), with the majority of carers over the age of 60 (n = 19).

A repeated measures design ('before and after') was used, measuring levels of knowledge, anxiety, depression, threat and self-efficacy (Halford 2002). Formal psychometric measures were used in the evaluation, including: the Dementia Quiz (Gilleard and Groom 1994), a 25-item multiple choice questionnaire with three subscales – biological (Biology), coping (Coping) and knowledge of services (Services); State-Trait Anxiety Inventory, STAI (Spielberger, Gorush and Lushene 1970); Centre of Epidemiologic Studies

Depression Scale, CES-D (Radolf 1977); Generalised Self-Efficacy Scale, GSES (Schwarzer and Jerusalem 1993); and the threat subscale from the Stress Appraisal Measure, SAM (Peacock and Wong 1990).

Table 16.1 shows the pre- and post-group mean scores for the measures used. Results indicated that, as a group, carers developed greater knowledge and self-efficacy and reported less anxiety, depression and perceived threat. However, the only statistically significant change was the increase in biological knowledge as measured by the subscale of the Dementia Quiz.

Table 16.1 Pre- and post-group mean scores (standard deviation) for 24 participant carers

		Pre-group (s.d.)	Post-group (s.d.)	Sig. (2-tailed)
Knowledge total		15.88 (5.2)	17.92 (2.9)	0.08
	Biology[1]	4.33 (2.1)	5.83 (1.3)	0.00*
	Coping[1]	5.79 (2.1)	6.75 (1.6)	0.06
	Services[1]	5.54 (2.0)	5.33 (1.0)	0.47
Self-efficacy[4]		28.54 (4.1)	30.04 (4.5)	0.09
Depression[3]		14.25 (10.6)	13.21 (9.3)	0.51
Anxiety				
	State[2]	40.96 (12.1)	37.71 (10.1)	0.10
	Trait[2]	40.46 (11.3)	40.08 (11.6)	0.83
	Threat[5]	13.54 (4.1)	12.13 (4.8)	0.12

*significant at the 0.01 level (2-tailed).
[1] Dementia Quiz subscales – biological (Biology), coping (Coping) and knowledge of services (Services): higher scores = greater knowledge.
[2] State–Trait Anxiety Inventory: higher scores = more anxiety.
[3] Centre of Epidemiologic Studies Depression Scale: lower scores = less depression.
[4] Generalised Self-Efficacy Scale: higher scores = greater self-efficacy.
[5] Threat subscale from the Stress Appraisal Measure: lower scores = less threat.

Very few psychosocial interventions have used anxiety measures to evaluate outcome for carers. Whilst some studies report no significant difference in informal caregivers' anxiety levels post-intervention (Lazarus *et al.* 1981; Wilkins *et al.* 1999), Millan-Calenti and colleagues (2000) reported a significant decrease in state anxiety but not trait anxiety. That is, the intervention used by Millan-Calenti and colleagues led to a reduction in carers' current levels of anxiety ('state' anxiety), but did not have an effect on their longstanding, pre-caring tendency to experience anxiety ('trait' anxiety). Results for the Positive Caring Programme are similar, but the small sample size means that the results were not statistically significant. Based on the effect sizes found in the Positive Caring Programme evaluation for the state anxiety change score (0.32) and total dementia knowledge scale (-0.41), it was estimated that a sample of 84 participants would be needed to demonstrate a statistically significant increase in levels of knowledge and reduced anxiety.

Example 2: BECCA Befriending Scheme

Befriending and Costs of Caring (BECCA) is a befriending scheme evaluated within a randomised controlled trial (see www.ncchta.org/project/ htapubs.asp, accessed 11 August 2008). The effectiveness of befriending schemes is unclear (Cattan et al. 2005), with one study on peer support for carers in the USA showing little measurable effect, with relationships lasting only a matter of months (Pillemer and Suitor 2002). Therefore, BECCA provides a welcome addition to the literature on long-term befriending for carers where the service was compared with 'support as usual' over a number of years. Here, befriending is defined as 'the provision of companionship and conversation', so focusing on emotional support. In this scheme, befriending is provided by trained befriending volunteers who commit to an hour per week for a minimum of six months. The befriending volunteers do not provide direct instrumental support or practical help to the carer, nor do they take the place of the carer, home care or nursing staff, as they do not provide any assistance for the person with dementia. Befrienders are not primarily information providers, but they are encouraged to 'signpost' carers to information and services as necessary.

The BECCA befriending scheme was initially set up in Norwich, UK, with an employed befriender facilitator based at the local volunteer bureau (Norwich and Norfolk Voluntary Services, NVS). NVS has appropriate public liability insurance and experience of managing other befriending projects, including a scheme for people with mental health problems and a scheme for people with physical disabilities. The scheme has now been extended to other parts of the county of Norfolk, in partnership with local branches of the Alzheimer's Society. In addition, two further schemes have been established within Age Concern, in the county of Suffolk and the London Borough of Havering, with part-time paid befriender facilitators based in Lowestoft, Ipswich and Harold Hill.

The paid befriender facilitators are responsible for the recruiting, screening, training and matching of volunteers, and the ongoing monitoring and support of befriender–carer relationships. The registration and screening procedure for volunteers includes use of a registration form, taking up of two references, and Criminal Records Bureau disclosures. All volunteers complete 12 hours of training, including: listening skills, stages of the befriending relationship, boundaries to the befriending role, carers' needs, understanding dementia and working safely in other people's homes. Training is supported by a written manual and carried out by the befriender facilitators in conjunction with other (usually local) trainers who have knowledge or expertise relevant to particular aspects of the training session.

Fourteen months after the first befriender facilitator came into post, there had been 68 expressions of interest from potential befriending volunteers, and six training courses had been held. Nine matches had been made with carers from a pool of 18 trained and screened befrienders. The first nine matched befrienders were predominantly female (seven of the nine) with a mean age of 65 (range 46 to 81 years). Many of these befrienders had previous experience as a carer, either of a family member or in a paid, non-family capacity. The befriended carers were also predominantly female (six wives of people with dementia, one husband, one daughter and one son), with a mean age of 68 (range 60 to 85). When asked to comment on their perception of the quality of the relationship with the befriender after one month, 67 per cent of carers rated the relationship as good or excellent. None of the carers expressed any concerns or complained of a poor relationship.

Case example – Charles and Judy

Charles had found his quality of life had diminished over the past three years since his wife, Judy, had started to develop signs of dementia. While they had both enjoyed taking part in the life of their small village for several years after Charles's retirement they had now almost become 'prisoners in their own home'. Many of their friends had either moved away, had difficulties of their own to deal with, or were unsure how to relate to them now that Judy had dementia. Charles and Judy were in contact with health and social services and Judy attended a day centre once a week, but Charles was feeling isolated. He would sometimes catch himself talking out loud and realise that he had not had a conversation with anyone for days.

Charles took part in the BECCA research project and was randomised to the intervention (befriending) arm of the trial. He met the befriender facilitator and was matched with a befriender from a small town some miles away from his home. The befriender arranged to visit Charles every other week, when Judy was at the day centre, and to talk on the phone during the weeks that they didn't meet. Charles had the opportunity to talk to someone in a way that he didn't feel free to do with his own family and this brought him great relief. In addition, little things would come up in conversation that made a big difference to the quality of both his life and also that of Judy – even though the befriender and Judy never met. For example, the befriender was able to signpost Charles to the voluntary driver scheme which provided assistance for people getting to hospital appointments, and also to the organisation that provided keys for disabled toilets. Charles was delighted as he had been getting concerned about the costs of taxis for hospital visits, and also he and his wife had declined going on trips as he wasn't able to assist her in public toilets. Soon Charles and his wife were once again able to enjoy trips out together.

Concluding remarks

The voluntary and charitable sectors provide a wealth of expertise in the support of interventions by volunteers, and in meeting differing social support needs of family carers. The support they provide can often be especially well tailored to individual circumstances and to local networks and communities.

Acknowledgements

The Positive Caring Programme was funded by a Lottery grant to the Eastern Region of the Alzheimer's Society, UK. The evaluation was carried out by Joanne Halford and supervised by Malcolm Adams. The evaluation, supported by the Alzheimer's Society, was approved by the University of East Anglia's Health Schools' Ethics Committee.

Fiona Poland and Georgina Charlesworth are part of the Befriending and Costs of Caring (BECCA) research team. The BECCA project (ISRCTN08130075), including the befriender facilitator posts, is funded by the Health Technology Assessment (HTA) Programme (project number 99/34/07). Befrienders' expenses are funded by Norfolk and Suffolk Social Services, the King's Lynn and West Norfolk branch of the Alzheimer's Society, and an ad hoc grant from the Department of Health to North East London Mental Health Trust. The views and opinions expressed in this chapter are those of the authors and do not necessarily reflect those of the Department of Health.

References

Barker, C. and Pistrang, N. (2002) 'Psychotherapy and social support: integrating research on psychological helping.' *Clinical Psychology Review 22*, 361–379.

Briggs, K. and Askham, J. (1999) *The Needs of People with Dementia and Those that Care for Them: A Review of the Literature.* London: Alzheimer's Society.

Cattan, M., White, M., Bond, J. and Learmouth, A. (2005) 'Preventing social isolation and loneliness among older people: a systematic review of health promotion interventions.' *Ageing and Society 25*, 41–67.

Cowen, E.L. (1982) 'Help is where you find it.' *American Psychologist 27*, 385–395.

Gilleard, C. and Groom, F. (1994) 'A study of two dementia quizzes.' *British Journal of Clinical Psychology 33*, 529–534.

Halford, J. (2002) 'An investigation into the relationship between knowledge of dementia and anxiety levels in informal caregivers looking after a person with dementia.' Thesis. School of Medicine, University of East Anglia.

Heller, K., Swindle, R.W. and Dusenbury, L. (1986) 'Component social support processes: comments and integration.' *Journal of Consulting and Clinical Psychology 54*, 466–470.

Hogan, B.E., Linden, W. and Najarian, B. (2002) 'Social support interventions: do they work?' *Clinical Psychology Review 22*, 381–440.

House, J.S. (1981) *Work Stress and Social Support.* Reading, MA: Addison-Wesley.

Kahn, R. and Antonucci, T.C. (1980) 'Convoys over the Life Course: Attachment, Roles and Social Support.' In P.B. Baltes and O.G. Brim (Editors) *Life-Span Development and Behavior*, Vol. 3. Orlando, FL: Academic Press.

Lazarus, L.W., Stafford, B., Coope, K., Cohler, B. and Dysken, M. (1981) 'A pilot study of an Alzheimer's patients' relatives discussion group.' *Gerontologist 21*, 353–358.

Millan-Calenti, J.C., Gandoy-Crego, M., Antelo-Martelo, M., Lopez-Martinez, M., Riveiro-Lopez, M.P. and Mayan-Santos, J.M. (2000) 'Helping the family carers of Alzheimer's patients: from theory to practice. A preliminary study.' *Archives of Gerontology and Geriatrics 30*, 131–138.

Milne, D.L. (1999) *Social Therapy: A Guide to Social Support Interventions for Mental Health Practitioners.* Chichester: Wiley.

Noon, J.M. (1999) *Counselling and Helping Carers.* Oxford: Blackwell.

Peacock, E.J. and Wong, P.T.P. (1990) 'The Stress Appraisal Measure (SAM): a multidimensional approach to cognitive appraisal.' *Stress Medicine 6*, 227–236.

Pillemer, K. and Suitor, J.J. (2002) 'Peer support for Alzheimer's caregivers: is it enough to make a difference?' *Research on Aging 24*, 171–192.

Radolf, L.S. (1977) 'The CES-D scale: a self-report depression scale for research in the general population.' *Applied Psychological Measurement 1*, 385–401.

Schwarzer, R. and Jerusalem, M. (1993) *Measurement of Perceived Self-efficacy: Psychometric Scales for Cross-Cultural Research.* Berlin: Freie Universität.

Spielberger, C.D., Gorush, R.L. and Lushene, R.E. (1970) *STAI Manual for the State-Trait Anxiety Inventory.* Palo Alto, CA: Consulting Psychologists Press.

Thoits, P.A. (1986) 'Social support as coping assistance.' *Journal of Consulting and Clinical Psychology 54*, 416–423.

Wilkins, S.S., Castle, S., Heck, E., Tanzy, K. and Fahey, J. (1999) 'Immune function, mood, and perceived burden among caregivers participating in a psychoeducational intervention.' *Psychiatric Services 50*, 747–749.

Further reading and related references

Charlesworth, G., Mugford, M., Shepstone, L., Wilson, E., Thalanany, M. and Poland, F. (2008) 'Does befriending by trained lay workers improve psychological well-being and quality of life for carers of people with dementia, and at what cost? A randomised controlled trial.' *Health Technology Assessment*, 12. Available at www.ncchta.org/project/htapubs.asp, accessed 11 August 2008.

Charlesworth, G., Shepstone, L., Wilson, E., Reynolds, S., Mugford, M., Price, D., Harvey, I. and Poland, F. (2008) 'Befriending carers of people with dementia.' *British Medical Journal*, 336(7656), 1295–1297.

Charlesworth, G., Tzimoula, X., Higgs, P. and Poland, F. (2007) 'Social networks, befriending and support for family carers of people with dementia.' *Quality in Ageing – Policy, Practice and Research 8*, 2, 37–44.

Hooper, E., Charlesworth, G., Poland, F. and Vaughan, S. (2004) 'Recruiting carers and befrienders: experiences from the Befriending and Cost of Caring (BECCA) study.' *Signpost 9*, 1, 7–10.

Knights, N., Tzimoula, X., Clarke, H., Bartlett, A. and Charlesworth, G. (2006) 'Loneliness and befriending.' *PSIGE – Psychology Specialists Promoting Psychological Wellbeing in Later Life Newsletter – 96*, 29–32. Available at www.psige.org/newsletters.php, accessed 11 August 2008.

List of Contributors

Emer Begley is a PhD student at Trinity College Dublin. She was the Irish research co-ordinator for the ENABLE project. Her research interests include the lived experience of dementia and social and health care policy.

Molly Burnham is a retired Occupational Therapist living in the south of England. She has a particular interest in the role of the occupational therapist in helping maintain the lifestyles of people with dementia and their families.

Suzanne Cahill is the Director of The Dementia Services Information and Development Centre at St James Hospital in Ireland and a Lecturer in Social Policy in Ageing at Trinity College Dublin. Her research interests include dementia and quality standards, assistive technology, family caregiving, and the assessment of dementia in primary care.

Inge Cantegreil-Kallen, PhD, is a Clinical Psychologist and researcher at the Department of Clinical Gerontology, Broca Hospital in Paris and INTERDEM co-ordinator for France. Her current interests are obstacles and facilitators in diagnosing dementia, disclosure of diagnosis, support interventions for caregivers and systemic family therapy in Alzheimer's disease.

Irene Carr is a Lecturer in Mental Health for Older People at the Institute of Health and Social Care, Guernsey. Her initial area of interest was psychosocial interventions in the early stages of dementia, but has now broadened to include a wide range of nurse/formal carer education regarding most aspects of dementia care. Her current research focus is superstition in dementia pertaining to Guernsey residents.

Georgina Charlesworth, PhD, is a Lecturer in Clinical and Health Psychology of Old Age at University College London and a Consultant Clinical Psychologist in the NHS, UK. Her research interests are in psychosocial interventions for family carers of people with dementia.

Rabih Chattat is Associate Professor of Clinical Psychology at the Faculty of Psychology, University of Bologna. His interests are in both psychosocial intervention with people with dementia and their caregivers, and in the training of practitioners.

Linda Clare, PhD, Professor in Psychology, is a Clinical Psychologist at the University of Wales Bangor. Her research interests focus on psychological understanding and intervention in cognitive impairment and dementia, including memory rehabilitation.

Richard Cheston is a Consultant Clinical Psychologist working for Avon and Wiltshire Mental Health Care Partnership Trust in England and Honorary Lecturer at Bath University. His main research interest concerns the development of psychosocial interventions based on an understanding of the experiences of people with dementia.

Jacomine de Lange is Senior Researcher at the Trimbos-institute, Netherlands Institute of Mental Health and Addiction and Associate Professor at the Institute for Health Care Studies, Rotterdam. Her interests are in research and education in care for older people and their carers and particularly in dementia care.

Jocelyne de Rotrou, PhD, is a Neuropsychologist at the Broca Hospital in Paris. Her current research interests are screening tests for dementia and psycho-educative programmes for dementia caregivers.

Rose-Marie Dröes, PhD, is Associate Professor responsible for the research programme Care and Support in Dementia at the Department of Psychiatry and the Alzheimer centre of the VU University medical centre in Amsterdam and the Regional Mental Health Care Institute GGZ-Buitenamstel Geestgronden in Amsterdam. Her research interests are the needs of people with dementia and their carers, development and effectiveness of psychosocial interventions (including support by means of information technology), and implementation of proven effective psychosocial interventions for people with dementia and their carers, such as the Meeting Centres Support Programme.

Manuel Franco is Head of Psychiatry, Department of Zamora Hospital, Spain. He is Associate Professor at Salamanca University and the Research and Development Director of the INTRAS Foundation. He is also Co-Director of Neuropsychologic Program of Salamanca, Spain.

Marie V. Gianelli is Associate Professor at the Faculty of Medicine and Surgery, University of Genova (Italy), a member of INTERDEM and a Consultant Psychologist for INRCA (Italian National Research Centre on Ageing). She is a clinical psychologist and her main interests are in clinical practice, research and training for practitioners on psychosocial approaches to dementia.

Gillian Gibson, RGN, BSc (Hons) Psychology, now retired, was a Project Psychologist at the Hull Memory Clinic from its inception in 1991.

Pablo Gomez, is Manager of the INTRAS Spain Foundation where he is the Director of European programmes.

Maud Graff, PhD, is a Researcher at the Alzheimer's Centre and Researcher at the Occupational Therapy Department of the Radboud University Medical Centre, Nijmegen. Her research interests are in the field of occupational therapy in older people with dementia and their primary caregivers, focusing on daily functioning and quality of life, and on caregiver competence and quality of life.

Inger Hagen, MSc (Chemistry), PhD (Faculty of Medicine, University of Oslo), started her own company in 1998. Based on experiences as family carer she has developed assistive aids for people with dementia to support time orientation and planning of daily activities.

Joanne Halford is a Chartered Clinical Psychologist working in her own private practice based in Kent and Surrey. Her specialist interests include neuro-rehabilitation, dementia carer stress and general adult mental health.

Jaswinder Harrison, Clinical Psychologist, has worked at Hull Memory Clinic, UK for over two years as a Clinical Psychologist. Her research interest are on the effects of personality on the adjustment to dementia in patients and their family members.

Hilary Husband is a Consultant Clinical Psychologist with the Norfolk and Waveney Mental Health Partnership Trust and Honorary Lecturer at the University of East Anglia, UK. Her research interests include professionals' communication skills and interventions in dementia.

Karen Jarvis received The Queen's Nursing Institute Award for Nursing and also a Health Action Zone Fellowship. These enabled her to develop work with people with dementia and their families. Karen is a Community Mental Health Nurse for Older People working with Humber Mental Health Teaching NHS Trust in Hull, England.

Kate Jones, PhD, is a Research Fellow at the Dementia Services Development Centre, University of Wales Bangor, supporting the Wales Dementias and Neurodegenerative Diseases Research Network (NEURODEM Cymru). She has contributed to a number of evaluation projects in dementia care, including a study of reminiscence work for people with dementia and their carers jointly.

Jill Manthorpe is Professor of Social Work and Director of the Social Care Workforce Research Unit at King's College London, UK. Her research interests include social care for older people and carers: covering risk, safeguarding, ethics and mental capacity.

Franka Meiland, PhD, is Senior Researcher at the Department of Psychiatry, VU University Medical Centre, and GGZ Buitenamstel Geestgronden in Amsterdam. Her research interests include psychosocial interventions and information technology solutions to support people with dementia and their carers: development, effect studies and implementation.

Esme Moniz-Cook, PhD, is Chair of INTERDEM, Professor of Clinical Psychology and Ageing at the Institute of Rehabilitation, University of Hull, UK and a Consultant Clinical Psychologist in the NHS, UK. Her interests are in clinical practice and research on timely psychosocial intervention in early dementia and challenging behaviour.

Marcel Olde Rikkert is Head of the Department of Geriatric Medicine, University Medical Centre Nijmegen, Director of Alzheimer Centre Nijmegen (ACN), Principal Investigator in the Nijmegen Centre for Evidence Based Practice, and member of the Board of the European Alzheimer' Disease Consortium. The Nijmegen Geriatric Research Programme focuses on clinical research in brain failure with age, and promotes trials, descriptive studies and development of research methods within the Alzheimer Centre Nijmegen.

Fiona Poland is a sociologist and Senior Lecturer in Therapy Research in the School of Allied Health Professions at the University of East Anglia. Her research interests include community-based research, carer and older people's support, and social networks.

Anne-Sophie Rigaud, MD, is Professor of Geriatrics, Head of the Department of Clinical Gerontology at the Broca Hospital in Paris. She is an INTERDEM member and also member of the European Alzheimer's Disease Consortium (EADC). Her research interests include vascular dementia, Alzheimer's disease and mild cognitive impairment.

Giancarlo Savorani, MD, Geriatrician, is responsible for the Psychogeriatrics Unit at the Division of Geriatric Medicine of S. Orsola-Malpighi University Hospital in Bologna, Italy. His main activities are in the assessment and treatment of people with dementia and their caregivers and developing and promoting memory training programmes for healthy older people.

Steffi Urbas is an Art Therapist based at the Alzheimer Therapiezentrum der Neurologischen Klinik Bad Aibling, Germany.

Willem van Tilburg, MD, PhD, is Emeritus Professor in Clinical Psychiatry at the VU University Medical Centre and retired Medical Director of the Regional Mental Health Care Institute GGZ-Buitenamstel Geestgronden in Amsterdam. As a head of the Department of Psychiatry of the VU University medical centre he was supervisor of the developmental and research project Meeting Centres Support Programme between 1992 and 2003.

Susan Vaughan was the Befriender Facilitator (Norfolk) for the Befriending and Costs of Caring (BECCA) Research Project from 2002 to 2006, and is now retired.

Myrra Vernooij-Dassen is Co-Chair of INTERDEM, a Medical Sociologist in the Centre for Quality of Care Research, Principal Investigator in the Nijmegen Centre for Evidence-Based Practice and Director of the Alzheimer's Centre, Nijmegen (ACN) of the Radboud University Medical Centre. Her research interests include quality of care, psychosocial interventions, collaboration with professionals, carer competence and family support.

Hannah Wilkinson, BSc (Hons) Psychology, is a Research and a Clinical Assistant Psychologist at the Hull Memory Clinic. Her interests are in promoting healthy active lifestyles in early dementia and also in the role of social participation group interventions and maintenance of well-being in early dementia.

Bob Woods is Professor of Clinical Psychology of Older People at the University of Wales Bangor, where he directs the Dementia Services Development Centre. His research interests relate to the evaluation of psychological interventions for people with dementia and their supporters.

Index

activity problems, difficulty initiating
  actions 61
Acton, G.J. 212
Adaptation-Coping Model 202–3
  see also stress–appraisal–coping
    model;
    stress–coping/adaptation
    theory
ADAS (Alzheimer's Disease
  Assessment Scale) 100
advice see guidelines; information
  giving
Age Concern Surrey 176
Age Exchange (London) 156
Aggarwal, N. 26
Albert, M. 87
alcohol 53
Allen, C.K. 111
Allen, K. 158
'Alzheimer's Café' 28
Alzheimer's Europe 23
Alzheimer's Society, Positive Caring
  Programme 223–6
Amieva, H. 90
AMPS (Assessment of Motor and
  Process Skills) 111, 112
Anderson-Hanley, C. 195
Aneshensel, C.S. 211
Antonucci, T.C. 222
anxiety management 21
aphasias 59
Archer, S. 176
Archibald, C. 176
Arkin, S.M. 77
art therapy interventions 146–54
  aims and rationale 147–8
  methods and practices 148–53
    connection with self and others
      148, 150–1
    expression without words
      148–50
    presenting self 153
    spontaneous actions and
      instincts 151–3
  see also collage work
Askham, J. 223
assessment frameworks for
  interventions 24
assistive technologies
  ENABLE study findings 121–30
  evaluation of devices 119–20
  see also memory aids

associative memory deficits 89
Astell, A. 88
autobiographical memory 22
  see also reminiscence therapies
Autobiographical Memory Interview
  (AMI) 168–9
autonomy and control measures 63

Bäckman, L. 66, 74, 77, 88, 96
Baddeley, A.D. 112, 168
Bailey, M. 46
Baker, S. 147
Ballard, C. 53
Bamford, C. 17
Barker, C. 223
Barthel Index 100
Barthel, D.W. 100
Bartlett, E. 175
Barton, J. 46, 138
Bassett, R. 22
Bauckham, P. 140, 156, 160, 165,
  175
Beavis, D. 15
BECCA Befriending Scheme 22,
  226–8
Beck, A.T. 47
befriending schemes 226–8
behaviour therapy 21
Belgium
  early diagnosis issues 19
  funding and service provisions 12
Benbow, S. 15
Bender, M. 26, 140, 156, 160, 165,
  175–7, 181
Bengtson, V.L. 213–14
Benham, L. 147
Berger, B 17
Bird, M. 18, 63, 75
Bjork, R.A. 94
Bjørneby, S. 116
Blackwell, A. 89
Blom, M. 28
Bond, J. 26
Bornat, J. 157
Bourgeois, M.S. 76
Bowler, J. 53
Bozoki, A. 87
brain structures and functions,
  potential deficit problems 59
Brandt, J. 73–4
Breda, J. 19, 23

Brenes, G. 63
Breuil, V. 86
Briggs, K. 223
Broca's area, potential deficit problems
  59
Brodaty, H. 14, 187, 195, 213
Brody, E.M. 100
Brooks, J.O. 96
Bruce, E. 156, 158–9, 161, 167
Brush, J.A. 75
Bryden, C. 136
Bryden-Boden, C. 20
Bucks, R. 88
Burgener, S.C. 17
Burgess, R. 26
Burns, A. 53, 136, 177, 180, 213
Butcher, J. 21
Butti, G. 95

Cahill, S. 121, 129
calendars, assistive devices 119–30
Cambridge Cognitive Examination for
  Mental Disorders (CAMCOG-R)
  100
Cameron, C. 14, 17
Cameron, M.H. 86, 90
Camp, C. 18, 63, 74–5, 75, 94
Campbell, A. 13
Campus, J. 28
Cantegreil-Kallen, I. 85, 87
Caregiver Burden Inventory (CBI)
  191–2, 193
carer needs
  assessment measures 191–2, 193,
    215, 224–5
  evidence-based studies 14
  see also family carers
carer-focused psycho-educational
  support groups 186–95
  see also Meeting Centres Support
    Programme
Caron, W.A. 195
Carver, C.S. 192
'cash for care' services 23
Cattan, M. 226
Centre for Epidemiological Studies
  Depression Scale (CES-D)
  224–5
Chambers, P. 176
change and dementia 213
Charlesworth, G. 46, 187

Cherry, K. 18, 63
Cheston, R. 46, 136, 141, 143, 170, 175
choice of interventions 24–6, 27–9
Christensen, H. 74
Cimetière, C. 85
Clare, L. 18, 22, 26, 46, 65, 73–8, 86, 90, 107, 175
Clarke, C. 15
Clinician's Global Impressions tool 100
Clock Drawing Test 100
co-working 139
Cochrane protocols and reviews, overview of interventions 35–6
Cockburn, J. 112
cognitive assessment tools 98, 100–1
cognitive behavioural therapy
    post diagnosis 46
        case example 46–8
cognitive focused interventions
    aims and tasks 30
    guidelines 30
    see also individual therapies
cognitive maps 58–60, 62
Cognitive Rehabilitation (CR) 21–2, 64, 73–8
    building on retained memory 74–6
    case examples 64–5
    compensating for problems 76
    guidelines 77
    implementing CR interventions 77
    see also GRADIOR (personalised computer-based CT programme)
'cognitive reserve' 18, 53, 82–3
Cognitive Stimulation Therapy (CST) 21–2, 81–90
    background and overview 81
    concept and definitions 82–5
    evidence-base (France) 85–6
    goals and methods 82–5
    session contents 84–5
    new directions 86–7
        developing programmes and frameworks 87–9
cognitive therapy 21
Cognitive Training (CT) 21
collage work 158–61, 163–4
compensation techniques (memory) 65, 76, 93–4
computer-aided rehabilitation 93–104
    background and evidence-base 93–7
    benefits 97
    problems and remedies 96–7
    control and autonomy measures 63
Cooke, D.D. 187
Coon, D.W. 187–9
coping with diagnosis 43–5
Coping Orientations to Problems Experienced (COPE) 192, 193
coping theory 202
Cossio, A. 147
cost benefit analysis 23

counselling services, post diagnosis 45–6
couple participation in group reminiscence 165–9
Cowen, E.L. 222
Crutch, S.J. 146
cues and prompts 65, 76
Cuijpers, P. 202
Cummings, J.L. 191, 204

Daly, T. 176
Dartigues, J.F. 90
Dautzenberg, M. 211
Davidson, K. 176
Davis, K.L. 100
de Boer, M.E. 19
de Klerk-Rubin, V. 175
de Rotrou, J. 82–7
delayed recall 85
    as predictor of dementia 88
dementia
    attitudes towards 16–20
    diagnosis 14–15, 17–20
Dementia Quiz 224–5
Dementia Voice Group Psychotherapy (DVGP) project 140–3
depression 176–8
Derksen, E. 219
DIADEM study 15–16, 18
diagnosis issues 14–15
    case example 46–8
    disclosure considerations 40–3
    disclosure rates 41–2
    fears and anxieties 43–5
    secrecy and concealment 44
    stigma concerns 17–20
    withholding information 40–1, 43
    see also support around diagnosis
diary-keeping 84, 94
Disch, R. 156
disclosure of diagnosis 40–3
    carer attitudes 42–3
    impacting on early intervention initiatives 54–5
    informing carers 42
    rates of disclosure 41–2
    timing problems 54
'double stigma' issues 15–16
Downs, M. 212
Driver, B. 147
Dröes, R.M. 202–3, 205
drug therapies 14–15
Dunkin, J. 195
Dusenbury, L. 223
'dysexecutive syndrome' 62

Eagger, S. 46, 138
early dementia, identification problems 14
early psychosocial interventions 20–3
    choice and selection frameworks 24–6, 27–9
    importance of evidence-base 13, 23

personalised approaches 23–6
    potential drawbacks, mood problems 51–2
    practice considerations 24–6
    protocols and programmes 55–6
        cognition-orientated activities 63–6
        information giving activities 56–62
        promoting control and pleasure 63
        promoting general health 62–3
        promoting social and pleasurable activities 66–7
        rationale for use 52–5
    types
        intensive communication methods 20
        signposting 20
        standard psychological therapies 21
        therapies to promote well-being 21–2
    see also support around diagnosis
educational sessions see group-based psycho-educational interventions
Edwards, A.B. 189
Eggermont, L. 53
Ellrodt, G. 211
ENABLE project 115–30
    background and aims 115–16, 117–18
    Irish context 117–21
        criteria for participation 118
        description of assistive technologies evaluated 119
        recruitment and selection of participants 120
        study findings and outcomes 121–30
Engelborghs, S. 53
'enhancing of neuronal reserves' 53
epidemiology of dementia, incidence and prevalence data 12
episodic memory 82
Epstein, C. 18
Erde, E. 43
errorless learning techniques 75
establishing supportive services
    aims and tasks 31
    guidelines 31
European comparisons
    epidemiological data 12
    funding and service provisions 12
    as models for practice 13–14
    stigma and attitudes 18–20
Everybody's Business (DoH 2005) 137
evidence-based studies, gaps in knowledge 13–14
executive function exercises 85
external memory aids 63–4
    see also assistive technologies

face recognition programmes 65
Falk, B. 147

falls prevention, information and advice 58, 61
family care giving needs *see* carer needs
family carers
  intervention planning 25
  participation in group sessions 165–9, 186–95
  peer support and befriending schemes 226–8
  pros and cons of early interventions 51–2
  psycho-educational interventions 186–95, 201–8, 211–20
family counselling programmes 22
Feil, N. 136
Felling, E. 214
Ferri, C. 116
Ferris, S. 89
Finnema, E. 67, 202
Fisher, M. 176
Flannery, R. 67
folic acid 53
Folkman, S. 187, 202
Folstein, M.F. 47, 100, 111, 191
Folstein, S.E. 47, 100, 111, 191
Forbat, L. 175
Ford, G.R. 195
France
  funding and service provisions 12
  use of cognitive stimulation therapies 81–90
Franco, M. 97, 103
free recall 88
Freeman, M. 100
Friedell, M. 20
From Grandmother with Love (Pettigren and Woodin 1992) 171
frontal lobes, potential deficit problems 59
funding for services
  as percentage of GDP 12
  as percentage of health budget 12
  see also resource allocation

Gallagher, C. 117
Gallagher-Thompson, D. 46, 136, 187
Garland, J. 140
Gaugler, J.E. 212
General Health Questionnaire 204
Generalised Self-Efficacy Scale (GSES) 225
Gerber, G.J. 181–2
Germany, use of art therapy with dementia 146–54
Gibson, F. 156, 167
Gibson, G. 54, 179
Gillard, J. 170
Gilleard, C. 224–5
Gilliard, J. 42, 52, 55, 141
Gillies, B. 17, 31
Gillon, R. 40
Gitlin, L. 52
goals of intervention *see* personal outcomes
Goffman, G.E. 16
Goldberg, D.P. 204

Goodman, C.C. 212
Gorush, R.L. 224–5
Gosselin, A. 86
Goudie, F. 136
GRADIOR (personalised computer-based CT programme) 93–104
  background and overview 93–7
  development 97–9
  methods and applications 99–102
    case examples 99–102
    modules and components 98
Grady, C. 53
Graff, M.J.L. 22–3
Graham, J.E. 22
Graham, N. 187
Grandparent's Book (Pedersen and Taylor-Smith 1995) 171
Green, A. 14, 187, 213
Grol, R. 219
Groom, F. 224–5
group CST (Cognitive Stimulation Therapy) 21
group-based interventions, general considerations and practical advice 26, 138–9, 166, 177–8
group-based memory therapies 106–13
  aims and rationale 107–8
  case examples 111–12
  content and course sessions 108–11
  selection of individuals 111–13
group-based psycho-educational interventions 186–95
  background and rationale 188–90
  context and overview 186–8
  methods and outcomes 190–4
group-based psychotherapy 21, 135–44
  general considerations 138–9
  person-centred care approaches 136–8
  study to evaluate effectiveness 140–3
    case examples 141–3
group-based reminiscence work 156–9, 165–9
  case examples 168–9
  guidelines 169–71
  practical considerations 166
  session contents 167
group-based support sessions *see* men's support groups
Guest, C. 191–2
guidelines
  for early diagnosis and recognition 19
  for life-story and collage work 169–71
  for memory CR interventions 77
Gwilliam, C. 42

Hachinski, V. 53
Hagen, I. 116–17
Haggerty, A. 137

Halford, J. 224
Hanley, I. 76
Happiness, Confidence and Affect self-rating scales 180
Harley, J.P.Y. 94
Hausman, C.D. 46
Hawkins, D. 46, 138
Haworth, D. 212
Heal, H.C. 42–3
health promotion initiatives 15, 18
  medication effects and falls prevention 53–4
  protocols and reviews 62–3
  see also group-based psycho-educational interventions
Hébert, R. 186–7, 195
Heller, K. 223
Heller, L. 15
Heller, T. 15
Henderson, A.S. 175
Herbert, R. 212
Hill, R.D. 66, 75
Hillier, V.F. 204
hobbies 61
Hock, C. 94
Hodgson, S. 156, 158–9, 165
Hoffman, M. 94
Hogan, B.E. 223
Holthe, T. 116
home-based interventions, early intervention studies 51
House, J.S. 222
The Hull Drop-in Memory Centre 166–72
The Hull Memory Clinic 55–67
  background and programme contexts 51–2
  illustrative case studies 58–62, 64–5, 67
  intervention rationale 52–5
  'prevention' and health promotion initiatives 53–4
  protocols and programmes
    basic overview 55–6
    cognition-orientated activities 63–6
    family carer support 62
    information giving activities 56–62
    promoting control and pleasure 63
    promoting general health 62–3
    promoting social and pleasurable activities 66
  specific activities
    face recognition programmes 65
    question and answer sessions 60–1
    use of cognitive maps 58–60, 62
    use of memory aids 63–4, 65
    use of Seattle Depression Protocol 66
    workshops for families 56–7, 67
Hultsch, D.F. 21, 24, 53

Husband, H.J. 42–4, 46

Iliffe, S. 14, 18–19, 175, 177, 212–13
implicit memory 82
in-home occupational therapy services 22, 23
incidence of dementia 12
individualised approaches 23–6, 202, 212–20
information giving
    use of cognitive maps 58–60, 62
    use of 'question and answer' sessions 60–1
    use of workshops 56–7
    see also group-based psycho-educational interventions
initiating activities, problems and difficulties 59, 61, 62
Innes, A. 23
intensive communication methods 20
Interactive Multimedia Cognitive Stimulation (IMCS) programmes 95–6
INTERDEM 23, 29, 32
interventions for early dementia see early psychosocial interventions
Ireland, funding and service provisions 12
Isaacs, R. 146
Italy
    funding and service provisions a 12
    use of carer-focused psycho-educational support groups 186–95
item locating devices 119–30

Jacoby, R. 177
Jagger, B. 159
James, A. 51
Jané-Llopis, E. 66
Jansen, A.P. 18
Jarvis, K. 158–9, 161, 169
Jerusalem, M. 225
Jeste, D, V. 104
Joling, K.J. 18, 22
Jones, K. 141, 170
Jonsson, L. 116
Josephsson, S. 75

Kahn, R. 222
Kang, J. 212
Karlsson, T. 75
Katsuno, T. 17
Keady, J. 15, 178
Kendrich, T. 212
Killick, J. 147, 158
Kipling, T. 46
Kitwood, T. 40, 107
Knapp, M. 23
Knight, B.G. 186–7

Kopelman, M. 168
Koschera, A. 14, 187, 213
Kosloski, K.D. 194–5
Kuypers, J. 213–14

LACLS (Large Allen Cognitive Level Screen) 111
Landauer, T.K. 94
De Lange, J. 202
Lavoie, J.P. 187
Lawrence, L. 158
Lawton Scale 100
Lawton, M.P. 100
Lazarus, L.W. 225
Lazarus, R.S. 187, 189, 202
Lees, K. 26, 175
Lévesque, L. 188
Levy, R. 177
Liberman, R.P. 189
Liebmann, M. 147
life review work 21, 158
    collage work 158–61, 163–4
    creating story books 159–63, 169–71
Linden, W. 223
link-making activities 75
Little, A.G. 74
Lobo, A. 100
locating lost items 119
Lodgson, R. 66
logical memory deficits 89
Lories, G. 97
Lushene, R.E. 224–5
Luszcz, M. 75
Lutzky, S.M. 186–7

McAfee, M. 137
McCabe, L. 23
McCurry, S.M. 66
McDaird, D. 186–7
McEvoy, C.L. 107
McHugh, P.R. 47, 100, 111, 191
McKitrick, L.A. 94
MacGregor, K. 147
Macijauskiene, J. 23
Macofsky-Urban, F. 186–7
Magni, E. 188
Mahony, F.I. 100
Malec, J.F. 94
The Man Who Mistook His Wife for a Hat (Sacks) 67
mandala drawings 150
Manthorpe, J. 14, 175, 177, 182, 212, 220
Marshall, A. 137
Marshall, M. 116
Marshall, V.W. 213
Mason, E. 175
Matthews, C.G. 94, 97
Meadows, G. 147
medication-induced problems, falls 54
Meeting Centres Support Programme 201–8
    background and rationale 201–3

criteria for inclusion 203
evaluation and research 203–4
implications for future research 207–8
methods and applications 204–7
case examples 206–7
memory activities
    cognitive rehabilitation 64–5, 73–8, 93–4
    elaborating information and link-making 75
    errorless learning techniques 75
    expanding rehearsal techniques 75, 76
    maximising cognitive strengths 65–6
    prophylactic cognitive rehabilitation 63–4
    use of computer-based techniques 93–104
    use of mnemonics 75
memory aids 63–4, 65, 76, 93–4
    see also assistive devices
memory assessments 98, 100–1
    post-test protocols 55–67
    selection for group therapies 111–12
    use of Autobiographical Memory Interview (AMI) 168–9
memory clinic studies 51–68
    background 51–2
    illustrative case studies 58–62, 64–5, 67
    intervention rationale 52–5
    'prevention' and health promotion initiatives 53–5
    protocols and programmes
        basic overview 55–6
        cognition-orientated activities 63–6
        family carer support 67
        information giving activities 56–62
        promoting control and pleasure 63
        promoting general health 62–3
        promoting social and pleasurable activities 66
    specific activities
        face recognition programmes 65
        question and answer sessions 60–1
        reminiscence with couples in group sessions 165–9
        use of cognitive maps 58–60, 62
        use of life story books 159–63, 169–71
        use of memory aids 63–4, 65
        use of the Seattle Depression Protocol 66
        use of collage work 158–61, 163–4
        workshops for families 56–7, 67
    timing of interventions 54–5

memory deficits
  in early dementia 74
    associative memory problems
      89
    delayed recall problems 88
    logical memory problems 89
    verbal fluency problems 88–9
    rehabilitative activities 64–5, 73–8
    building on remaining memory
      74–6
    compensating for problems 76
Memory Diary (Short 1993) 171
memory group therapy 106–13
  aims and rationale 107–8
  case examples 111–12
  content and course sessions
    108–11
  selection of individuals 111–13
memory lapses, and anxiety 44
memory training 73–8
  computer-assisted programmes
    93–104
  problems and remedies 96–7
men's support groups 174–84
  background and rationale 174–6
  developing gender specific groups
    178–84
Meyers, B.S. 41
Miesen, B.M.L. 28
Mild Cognitive Impairment (MCI)
  21–2
  four 'at risk' functional domains
    88
  'prevention' strategies 53–5
  use of cognitive stimulation
    (CS) 81–90
Millan-Calenti, J.C. 225
Mills, M. 175
Milne, D.L. 223
Mini Cognitive Examination 100
Mini Mental State Examination
  (MMSE) 100, 140, 191
Mitchell, R. 147
Mittelman, M.S. 18, 22, 195
mneumonics 75
Mohs, R.C. 100
Moise, P. 15
Moniz-Cook, E.D. 16–18, 21, 22,
  24, 27–9, 30–1, 51–67, 158,
  170, 172, 179, 213
Montgomery, R.J.V. 194–5
mood assessment tests 100, 180
  for carers 191–2, 193, 224–5
mood problems
  and early interventions 51–2
  use of gender-specific support
    groups 176–84
  use of psychosocial group therapies
    135–44
Moos, R.H. 202
Moriarty, J. 220
Moss, P. 14, 17
Moyes, M. 158–9, 161, 165
Müller-Spahn, F. 94
Murphy, C. 156–9, 161, 165, 182
Murray, J. 186–7
My Life Story (Short 1993) 171

Nadal, E. 43
Naidoo, J. 52, 55
Najarian, B. 223
National Dementia Strategy 15
Neal, D. 147, 158
Neely, A.S. 66
Netherlands
  family counselling programmes 22
  funding and service provisions 12
  in-home occupational therapy 22
  primary care case management 18
neuro-protective measures 53
Neuropsychiatric Inventory (NPI)
  191, 193, 204
newspaper reviews 84
NICE/SCIE guidelines (2006) 19
Nicholson, L. 29
night lights, automatic devices
  119–30
Nobili, A. 188
Nolan, M. 178
Noon, J.M. 223
normalisation and social integration
  measures 63
Norris, A. 140, 156, 160, 165, 175
Novak, D.H. 40
Novak, M. 191–2
Nutbeam, D. 52, 54

occipital lobes, potential deficit
  problems 59
occupational therapy services,
  home-based interventions 22, 23
O'Connor, D.W. 213
Oken, D. 40
Olin, J.T. 100
Oliver, D. 54
Onder, G. 21, 30
Opie, J. 213
Orani, M. 63
O'Reilly, S. 117
orientation activities 63–4, 84
Ory, M.G. 188–9
O'Shea, E. 117
Otteson, O.J. 195

Page, S. 15
Palmer, K. 88
Panza, V. 94
Parahoo, K. 13
parietal lobes, potential deficit
  problems 59
Parker, J. 147
Pattee, J.J. 195
Patterson, R.L. 107
Patton, M. 124
Paykel, E.S. 189
Peacock, E.J. 225
Pearce, A. 175
Pearlin, L.I. 214
Pedersen, J. 171
peer support and befriending schemes
  226–8
Penhale, B. 157

person-centred care, and group
  interventions 136–8
personal outcomes 24–5
personalised psychosocial
  interventions 23–6, 202,
  212–13
  Primary Carer Support Programme
    211–20
Persoon, J.M.G. 214
Petersen, R. 86
Pettigren, J. 171
Piccolini, C. 107
Pierzchala, A. 18
Pillemer, K. 226
Pinquart, M. 63
Pistrang, N. 175, 223
planning support interventions 25–6
A Pocket Book of Memories (Sheppard
  and Rusted 1999) 171
Portugal
  early diagnosis issues 19
  funding and service provisions 12
Positive Caring Programme 223–6
Pratt, R. 26, 28
prevalence of dementia 12
'prevention' strategies 53–5
Price, E. 182
Primary Carer Support Programme
  211–20
  background and rationale 211–14
  evidence and theoretical basis
    213–14
  methods and applications 214–19
    case examples 216–18
problem-solving activities 85
Procter, L. 51
prompts and cues 65, 76
prophylactic cognitive rehabilitation
  63–4
protocols for intervention 55–6
psychological and social support
  aims and tasks 30–1
  guidelines 30–1
psychosocial interventions for early
  dementia *see* early psychosocial
  interventions
psychotherapeutic group work *see*
  group-based psychotherapy
public awareness campaigns 19–20
public health promotion initiatives *see*
  health promotion initiatives
Purandare, N. 53, 63
Pusey, H. 187
Pynoos, J. 212

Quality of Life and Management of
  Living Resources programmes
  115
Quayhagen, M. 77
Quayhagen, M.P. 77
'question and answer' sessions 60–1
Quinn, R. 18

Rabins, P. 213
Radolf, L.S. 225

Rainsford, C. 26, 175
Randeria, L. 26
reality orientation *see* Cognitive
    Stimulation Therapy (CST)
recall techniques 84
Reever, K.E. 51
rehearsal techniques 94
rehearsing activities 75
Reifler, B.V. 177
relaxation therapies 21
'Remembering Yesterday, Caring
    Today' reminiscence project 156
reminiscence therapies 22, 156–72
    background and overview 156–9
    collage work 158–60, 163–4
    couples participation in group
        sessions 165–9
    life story books 159–63, 169–71
repetition and dementia 151
repetitive practice techniques 94
reserve capacity theories *see* 'cognitive
    reserve'
resource allocation
    competing approaches 15, 23
    cost benefit analysis 23
respite care 201–2, 212, 219
Reynolds, D. 15
Rice, K. 42
Rich, J.B. 73–4
Richards, D. 187
Richards, K. 52, 158–9, 170
Ridley, C. 147
Rivermead Behavioural Memory Test
    (RBMT) 112
Robertson, I. 97
Romero, B. 146–7
Rosen, W.G. 100
Rosewarne, R. 213
Rossor, M.N. 146
Roth, M. 100
Rowlands, J. 18
Russell, V. 51
Rusted, J. 171
Ruxton, S. 178

Sabat, S. 52
Sabin, N. 51
Sacks, O. 67
Sahakian, B. 89
Sainsbury, L. 179
Sandman, C.A. 77
Scheier, M.F. 192
Scherder, E. 53
Schneider, L.S. 100
Scholey, K. 136
Schooler, A. 214
Schreiber, L.S. 94
Schulz, R. 188–9
Schwarzer, R. 225
Schweitzer, P. 22, 156–9, 165, 168
Scoltock, C. 13
Scott, A. 175
Scott, J. 26
The Seattle Depression Protocol 66
secrecy and concealment 44

selecting interventions *see* choice of
    interventions
semantic categorisation techniques 84
Senesi, B. 189
Seron, X. 97
service interventions for early
    dementia *see* early psychosocial
    interventions
service provisions
    specialist medical professionals 12
    see also establishing supportive
        services
Sheppard, L. 147, 171
Shipway, E. 158
Short Sense of Competence
    Questionnaire (SSCQ) 215
Short, P. 171
Sica, C. 192
SIGN (Scottish Intercollegiate
    Guidelines Network) 19
signposting 20
Simon, C. 212
Sinason, V. 136
Sitzer, D.I. 104
Skowronski, J.J. 22
Smartbrain (IMCS programme) 95–6,
    102
Smits, C.H.M. 24
Snyder, L. 139, 176
social activities 61
    dealing with embarrassment 61
    dealing with 'shame' feelings 44
    normalisation and integration
        measures 63
social support theory 222–3
Social Therapy (Milne) 223
Solomon, K. 46
spaced retrieval techniques 63–4, 75,
    94
Spain
    early diagnosis issues 19
    funding and service provisions 12
spatial orientation activities 84
Spector, A. 53, 81, 86
Spielberger, C.D. 224–5
'spoiled identity' concepts 17
State-Trait Anxiety Inventory (STAI)
    224–5
Stern, Y. 18
Stevens, A.B. 75
stigma issues 15–16
    constructs and concepts 16–17
    current attitudes and approaches
        17–20
    European comparisons 18–20
Stokes, G. 136, 163, 170
Stress Appraisal Measure (SAM) 225
stress–appraisal–coping model 214
stress–coping/adaptation theory
    187–8
    see also Adaptation-Coping Model
strokes 60-1
Suitor, J.J. 226
supplements *see* vitamins and
    supplements
support around diagnosis 39–48
    aims and tasks 30

disclosure issues and concerns
    40–3
    guidelines 30
    individual coping strategies 43–5
    potential interventions 45–8,
        51–67
support measures *see* carer-focused
    psycho-educational support
    groups; Meeting Centres
    Support Programme; men's
    support groups; support around
    diagnosis
Sweep, M.A.J. 116
Swindle, R.W. 223
Szwabo, P. 46

Takahasi, K. 63
Talking About Memory Coffee Club
    28
Tamura, J. 63
targeting frameworks for intervention
    27–9
Tárraga, L. 95, 102
Taylor-Smith, A. 171
telephones, assistive devices 119–30
temporal lobes, potential deficit
    problems 59
temporal orientation activities 84
Teri, L. 22, 26, 46, 53, 66, 136, 177
Thoits, P.A. 223
Thommesen, B. 195
Thompson, A. 28
Thompson, C.P. 22
Thompson, L.W. 46, 187
Thrower, C. 137
TIA's (transient ischaemic attacks)
    60–1
time keeping, assistive devices
    119–20
Tokoro, M. 63
Topo, P. 116
'tribal stigma' 16–17
Truax, P. 66
Tsu, V.D. 202
Tuokko, H.A. 21, 24, 53
Twamley, E.W. 104
Tyler, J. 147

Validation therapy 136
van Dijkhurzen, M.I. 175
van Hout, H. 212
van Tilburg, W. 202, 205
vascular risk factors 53
Vassilas, C.A. 42
verbal fluency deficits 88–9
Verhey, F. 88
Vernooij-Dassen, M. 12, 14–15, 16,
    18, 22, 172, 188, 202, 211,
    213–15, 218
Versey, R. 89
Vidal, J.C. 86
Visser, P. 88
visual hallucinations 67
visual and verbal cues 65, 76

Vitamin C 53
vitamin E 53
vitamins and supplements,
    neuro-protective 53
voluntary sector interventions 222–8
  Positive Caring Programme 223–6

Walker, W.R. 22
Waller, D. 147, 159
Waring, J. 26, 175
Warner, M. 13
Warner, N. 42
Watkins, B. 141–3
websites, overview of interventions 35
Weintraub, J.K. 192
Wenger, C. 174–5
Wenz, M. 146–7
Wernicke's area, potential deficit
    problems 59
White, V. 175
Wilcock, J. 212
Wilkins, S.S. 225
Williamson, G.M. 188
Willis, J. 52, 55
Wilson, B.A. 74, 112, 168
Wilson, P. 147
Wimo, A. 116
Win, T. 54
Winblad, B. 116
Wind, A. 19
withholding information 40–1, 42–3
Wong, P.T.P. 225
Woodin, M. 171
Woods, B. 13, 156
Woods, R.T. 18, 24, 46, 66, 74,
    76–7, 107, 136, 158–9, 170,
    220
Woolham, J. 116
workshops for families 56–7
World Health Organization 158
worries and fears, at diagnosis 43–4

Yale, R. 46, 137
Yalom, I.D. 143

Zanetti, M. 86–7
Zanetti, O. 75, 188, 195
Zarit, J.M. 51
Zarit, S.H. 25–6, 51, 189